S0-DUM-219

OXFORD MEDICAL PUBLICATIONS

Tendinitis: its etiology and treatment

# Tendinitis: its etiology and treatment

## William D. Stanish
*Associate Professor of Surgery, Halifax, Canada*

## Sandra Curwin
*Associate Professor and Director of Physical Therapy, Husson College, Bangor, USA*

## and

## Scott Mandel
*Research Fellow, Orthopaedic and Sports Medicine Clinic of Nova Scotia, Canada*

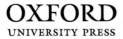

OXFORD
UNIVERSITY PRESS

*This book has been printed digitally and produced in a standard specification
in order to ensure its continuing availability*

# OXFORD
UNIVERSITY PRESS

Great Clarendon Street, Oxford OX2 6DP

Oxford University Press is a department of the University of Oxford.
It furthers the University's objective of excellence in research, scholarship,
and education by publishing worldwide in

Oxford New York

Auckland Cape Town Dar es Salaam Hong Kong Karachi
Kuala Lumpur Madrid Melbourne Mexico City Nairobi
New Delhi Shanghai Taipei Toronto
With offices in
Argentina Austria Brazil Chile Czech Republic France Greece
Guatemala Hungary Italy Japan South Korea Poland Portugal
Singapore Switzerland Thailand Turkey Ukraine Vietnam

Oxford is a registered trade mark of Oxford University Press
in the UK and in certain other countries

Published in the United States
by Oxford University Press Inc., New York

ISBN  0-19-263258-2

Printed and bound by CPI Antony Rowe, Eastbourne

# Contents

Introduction                                              1

1 Normal tendon                                           3

2 Etiology of tendinitis                                 19

3 Exercise and the muscle-tendon unit                    33

4 Achilles tendinitis                                    49

5 Jumper's knee                                          65

6 Humeral epicondylitis                                  83

7 Other tendinitides                                     99

8 Clinical results                                      117

References and bibliography                             125

Index                                                   135

# Introduction

Tendon, like other soft tissues, is susceptible to injury from a variety of sources: direct blows, excessive tensile force, even breaks or tears. The body's response to any injury is the 'inflammatory response', followed by repair. Tendinitis is the word used to describe inflammation of the tendon.

A newer concept is emerging in the discussion of chronic tendon disorders—tendinosis. It refers to a degenerative condition of the tendon that seems to be related to both age of the patient and activity level. Histologically, surgical specimens show very few inflammatory cells and are more likely to show degeneration, which can have fatty mucoid or hyaline features. Degenerative changes have also been seen in asymptomatic tendons (Kannus and Jozsa 1991), suggesting that normal forces across an abnormal tendon may play a role in the etiology of chronic tendon problems in older patients.

Inflammatory response to trauma seems most prevalent in tenosynovium and peritenon, giving rise to another new term—'peritendinitis' (literally, inflammation in the tissues around the tendon).

These terms can be confusing to separate for diagnostic purposes and it is easier to understand them as points on a continuum rather than discrete clinical entities. Throughout this book, the term 'tendinitis' is used to describe this continuum. Where a specific patients' injury lies on the continuum (and their treatment) will be influenced by variables such as patient age, duration of symptoms, and activity level. In general, older patients with long standing symptoms and a history of repetitive activity of that limb will be more likely to have tendinosis (with or without associated peritendinitis). In contrast, young patients with acute onset of symptoms will be more likely to have a true peritendinitis, without much associated tendon degeneration. Tendinitis occurs when the tendon bears more load than it can withstand repeatedly. It is at this point that damage and its sequelae inflammation and degeneration occurs. This can be due to excessive high loads across normal tendons or normal loads across degenerative tendons.

The word 'repeatedly' should be considered. It is known that a tendon can bear much more than the physiologic loads across it in daily use. Thus, acute failures of tendon are rare, as the ultimate tensile strength of tendon is not exceeded. Ultimate tensile strength can be defined as the stress needed to cause failure of a material in one loading cycle, in the case of tendon the force needed to pull the tendon apart. 'Why then do tendons become injured?' They become injured because the fatigue limit (or endurance limit) of the tendon is reached with repeated use. Repetitive loading of a material (tendon) will cause it to fail, even if loads are less than the ultimate tensile strength. This is illustrated by the example of the tab on a pop can breaking, after it is wiggled back and forth a few times. Thus, repeated stressful use (or 'overuse') of tendons causes damage to the internal architecture of the tendon, setting the stage for clinical symptoms. Most tendon injuries fall into the classification known as 'overuse syndrome'. Also, because tendons have less rich blood supply than other soft tissues such as skin or muscle they are slower in healing.

# 1   Normal tendon

Tendon structure determines its response to the tasks imposed on it during activity, so the normal tendon, its structure, function and metabolic activity, as well as its response to aging, activity, and immobility are considered first. Both the ultra-structure of the tendon and other structural factors, such as length and cross-sectional area, affect the way tendons behave when forces are applied to them. Blood supply and metabolic activity affect the rate of healing after injury, and changes due to aging, immobility, and activity affect the incidence of injury and its response to treatment. Since all these things influence the clinical course of tendinitis, this chapter lays the ground work for later discussion of tendinitis and its treatment.

## The muscle-tendon unit

Tendons are rope-like structures that connect muscles to bone. The muscles are the prime movers of the body—they contract and produce force. Tendons allow precise application of this force to the limb being moved. Thus, we speak of the muscle-tendon unit or a muscle and its attached tendon/tendons.

Muscles vary greatly in size, shape, and complexity (Fig. 1.1). Some are broad and flat, with wide, short tendons such as the gluteus maximus or rectus abdominis. Others, such as the fusiform biceps, have smaller, rounded, cord-like tendons. In general, the shorter and broader tendons are associated with muscles that create high levels of force, while longer and narrower tendons are associated with muscles that make precision movements, such as those seen in the hand (Jozsa and Kannus 1997). Although muscle and tendon are structurally separate, functionally they are one unit—the muscle-tendon unit. Thus it is unrealistic to consider and discuss tendon in isolation from its accompanying muscle, and we encourage the reader to bear this in mind throughout the following pages.

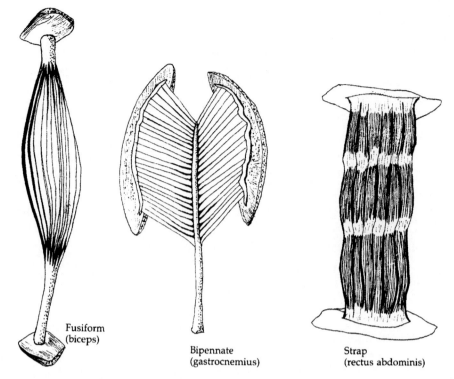

Fusiform
(biceps)

Bipennate
(gastrocnemius)

Strap
(rectus abdominis)

**Fig. 1.1  The appearance of three different types of muscle found in the body.**

## Structure

The composition and properties of tendon are very similar to those of other soft tissues such as ligaments, joint capsule and interosseous membranes, and fascia. All of these supply tensile strength, combined with flexibility. They are all collagen-based structures with relatively little cellularity, as compared to organs such as the liver or kidneys. The difference lies in the fact that all these structures, except fascia, connect bone to bone; while tendon is interspersed between muscle and bone. Other features unique to tendons are synovial sheaths and bursae. These act as friction reducing devices to help improve the efficiency of movement and decrease wear on tendons.

The insertion of tendon into bone involves a gradual transition from tendon to fibrocartilage, to mineralized fibrocartilage, to lamellar bone; similar to ligament insertion into bone. The presence of fibrocartilage means very few blood vessels traverse the bone-tendon junction. The junction between muscle and tendons is via projections of the tendon fibrils into the muscle membrane at the ends of the fasciculi (Viidik 1973). The infolding of the muscle membrane creates finger-like projections that interdigitate with the collagen fibres of the tendon, increasing the surface area of contact by up to as much as twenty times (Tidball 1991); similar to villi in the gastrointestinal tract. This increased area helps to dissipate force at the muscle-tendon junction, as seen in the animal studies of Eisenberg and Milton (1984) and Kvist *et al.* (1991).

## Ultrastructure

Tendon is composed mainly of collagen, being anywhere from 65–85% of its dry weight. It is embedded in a proteoglycan—water matrix or gel. The usual distribution is 30% collagen and 58–70% water. Elastin, another protein, is present in very small amounts (2%). These substances are produced by cells called fibroblasts that are found throughout the tendon, and become more numerous when connective tissue must be produced such as during development or an injury repair.

Collagen synthesis parallels that of other protein molecules. Amino acids are assembled into chains that fold into a triple helix (procollagen). As the triple helices leave the cell, enzymes in the extracellular environment remove part of the procollagen molecule; then it is known as tropocollagen. The tropocollagen molecule is considered the most fundamental unit in collagenous structures.

Present knowledge suggests that five tropocollagen units join to form a larger fibrous entity, the microfibril. The molecules are assembled in a staggered fashion, with each overlapping its neighbours by approximately 1/4 of its length (Fig. 1.2).

Next the microfibrils group into subfibrils, which in turn form fibrils—the basic load bearing units of ligaments or tendons. The collagen fibrils appear cross-striated, or banded, under the electron microscope because of the staggering of the tropocollagen molecules and gaps in the head-to-tail arrangement of the molecules.

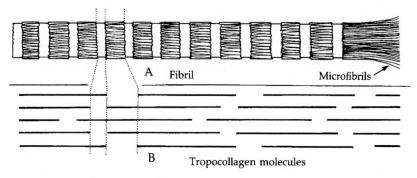

**Fig. 1.2 The staggering of tropocollagen molecules to form microfibrils and fibrils.**

Groups of parallel fibrils, surrounded by the matrix, are known as fibres. These may be as long as the tendon itself, and they associate into larger groups (primary tendon bundles), which then aggregate into fascicles. Surrounding the fascicles is a sheath (the endotenon), through which nerves and blood vessels run. These fascicles are the smallest collagenous structures that can be mechanically tested (Butler *et al.* 1978). Fibroblasts are found inside the fascicles, between the primary fibre bundles. Groups of fascicles surrounded by a second sheath called the epitenon, form the tendon proper. Outside the epitenon is a third sheath, the paratenon. Small amounts of fluid between the epitenon and the paratenon provide lubrication, preventing friction and damage to the tendon.

This complicated structure has been described by Kastelic *et al.* (1978) who termed it the 'hierarchical organization of tendon' (Fig. 1.3). The fibres and

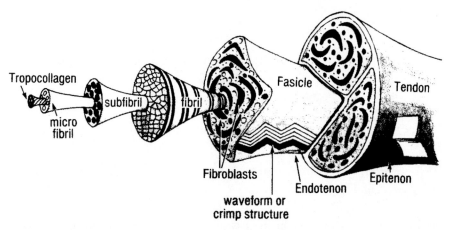

**Fig. 1.3 The hierarchical organization of the tendon, showing the various stages from molecule to tendon. Redrawn with permission from Kastelic, J., Galeski, A., and Baer, E. The multicomposite structure of tendon.** *Connect. Tissue Res.,* **6, 11–23, 1978.**

primary fibre bundles were not described by these authors, although they have been by others, reflecting the lack of agreement about tendon's structure. The fibres and primary fibre bundles reside between the fibril and fascicle level.

The collagen fibrils, though they are arranged longitudinally, are not straight; they appear to be zig-zag or crimped (Fig. 1.4). This may be due to either the transverse mechanical interaction between fibrils or buckling caused by shrinking of the intrafibrilar matrix with age. This wavy configuration, a characteristic feature of tendon, disappears when the tendon is stretched.

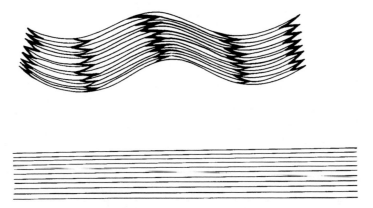

**Fig. 1.4 The collagen fibrils appear wavy when relaxed, but lose this crimped appearance when stretched.**

## Blood supply

Tendon is described in many textbooks as an avascular tissue in explanation of its slow rate of healing, however it is avascular only relative to tissue such as muscle and skin.

Most authors seem to agree that tendon receives its blood supply via three routes (although this agreement does not extend to the relative importance of each): the musculotendinous junction; along the length of the tendon; and the bone-tendon junction. Musculotendinous and tendon bone vessels are responsible for the distal thirds of the tendons respectively, while the vessels from the paratenon or synovial sheaths supply the central third.

### The musculotendinous junction

A number of longitudinal vessels traverse the musculotendinous junction, but these are found only in the superficial covering of the muscle (perimysium). The capillary circulation of muscle and tendon is completely separate, in keeping with the lack of continuity between the muscle and tendon fibres. The capillaries adjacent to the musculotendinous junction loop back into the muscle or tendon and there is no anastomosis between them. There are, however, small vessels that divide near the musculotendinous junction and supply branches to both muscle and tendon.

## The length of the tendon

The blood supply is from either paratenon (the thin filmy layer of areolar tissue covering the tendon) or the synovial sheath (which replaces the paratenon where the tendon is subjected to friction). The paratenon contains many vessels which are largely responsible for the tendon's blood supply, particularly (perhaps even solely) the middle third. Small branches from vessels in the peritenon run transversely towards the tendon and branch several times before assuming a course parallel to the tendon's long axis. Where tendons are invested with a synovial sheath, the paratenon continues between two layers of synovial tissue, as the mesotenon. The mesotenon provides access for the arteries, veins, and nerves through the synovial sheath and into the tendon. The mesotenon is also known as the vincula. The synovial fluid, produced by synovial cells lining the tendon sheath, also plays a role in the nutrition of sheathed tendons (Matthews 1976; Lundborg 1976).

Many authors ascribe great importance to the blood supply along the length of the tendon and relay the incidence of tendinitis to zones of decreased vasculature. This is one of the proposed etiologic factors in supraspinatus tendinitis of the shoulder (MacNab 1973), and it has been implicated in Achilles tendinitis as well (Smart et al. 1980; Clancy 1982). Since the rate of healing is affected by blood flow and much of the tendon appears to be solely dependent on this source of blood supply, this may be an important etiologic factor.

## The tendon-bone junction

The vessels of tendon and bone do not communicate directly because the tendon fibres gradually convert to fibrocartilage near the osseotendinous junction. There are, however, indirect anastomoses between tendon vessels and those of the periosteum. This source of blood supply provides up to one third of the tendon's requirements.

## Internal vasculature

The blood vessels within the tendon are orientated primarily longitudinally in the endotenon and thus are arranged around the fascicles. These vessels, arteriolar in size, are flanked by two veins. Capillaries loop from the arterioles to the venules but do not penetrate the collagen bundles. The internal system, aligned in the tendon's long axis, is fed by vessels in the epitenon which branch and enter the tendon radially, via the endotenon.

The vasculature of the tendon is variable and is reduced in areas of friction, torsion, compression, or excessive wear. This and its relationship to tendinitis is discussed further in Chapter 2.

## Innervation of tendon

The nerve supply to the tendon is sensory and is derived from the appropriate overlying nerve. Its branches infiltrate the tendons similar to blood vessels, although many of the nerve fibres end on the surface of the tendon. Normally, proprioceptive information is picked up via sensory nerve endings near the musculotendinous junction, and is relayed to the central nervous system. There are three types of mechanoreceptors: Ruffini corpuscles (slow adapting pressure sensors), Pacini corpuscles (fast adapting velocity sensors), and Golgi tendon organs (GTO), which are tension receptors similar to muscle spindles. There are also free nerve endings which function as pain receptors and are abundant in peritendinous tissue. The Golgi tendon organ responds primarily to tension within the tendons such as that produced during muscle contraction or passive stretch. The corpuscles respond to stimuli transmitted via the surrounding tissue, such as pressure, which also may be produced by muscle contraction. Since the amount of pressure depends on the force of the contraction, the lamellated corpuscles may provide more finely tuned feedback.

## Mechanics and function

The mechanical behaviour of a tendon depends on its structure. Its function is to transmit forces from muscle to bone. Since muscle produces force only when it is contracting, this has a stretching effect on the tendon, known in mechanical circles as a tensile force. Other types of force, such as compressive and shear, may also be applied to the soft tissues (Fig. 1.5).

Tendon withstands tensile forces well, better than bone in fact. Tendon resists shear forces less well and provides little resistance to compressive forces. Bone withstands compression much better than tension. Tendons must be flexible to allow unhindered movement and redirection of force 'around corners'. For example, the extensor pollicis longus passes around the radial tubercle, runs underneath the extensor retinaculum, and finally inserts on the distal phalanx of the thumb (Fig. 1.6). Note that the tendon is surrounded by a synovial sheath to reduce friction.

The tensile force applied to the tendon is resisted mainly by the collagen, which is characterized by poor elasticity but great mechanical strength.

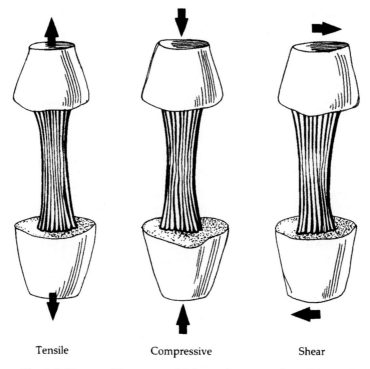

Tensile          Compressive          Shear

**Fig. 1.5 Types of force to which tendons may be subjected**

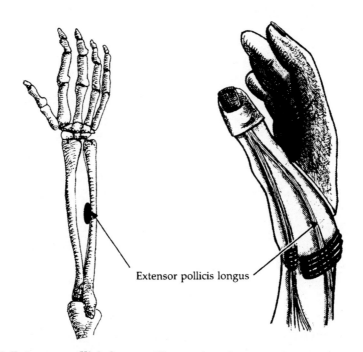

Extensor pollicis longus

**Fig. 1.6 Extensor pollicis longus, illustrating the curved paths that muscle-tendon units sometimes follow between origin and insertion.**

Because the collagen fibres are crimped, the initial response to tensile force is straightening of the fibres so that these waves, or crimps, disappear. Greater loads stress the fibrils themselves. The typical response of tendon to applied tensile force is shown in Fig. 1.7. The initial concave portion of the curve (Region I) is called the toe region. Under the conditions represented by this part of the curve, little force is required to elongate the tissue since the fibrils are straightening. This portion of the curve is felt to be governed by shearing within the matrix. The return of the crimp in the fibres after the force has been released in the toe region has been suggested to be due to the elastin present in the tendon. As more force is applied, the fibrils straighten and the force–time curve becomes linear, which means that greater magnitudes of force are necessary to elongate the tendon. As more force is applied, some fibres begin to fail (in Region III). This, of course, increases the load on those fibres that remain intact and more and more fibres rupture. As this happens, the tendon bears less load although it may or may not be completely ruptured at this point.

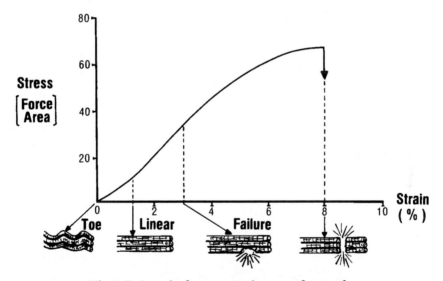

Fig. 1.7 A typical stress-strain curve for tendon.

## Size

The same is true for both muscle and tendon: the more fibres present, or the larger those fibres, the more force the tendon can withstand. Thus, there is a direct correlation between cross-sectional area and applied load (Fig. 1.8). Increased size means that the tendon is more resistant to stretch—that it is

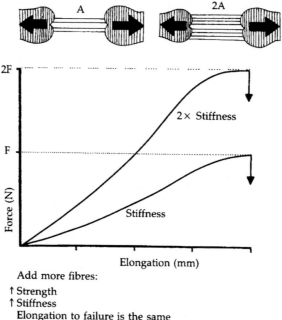

Add more fibres:

↑ Strength
↑ Stiffness
Elongation to failure is the same

**Fig. 1.8 The effect of area on tendon behavior. Note that the larger tendon is 'stiffer'; that is more force is borne per unit of elongation. Redrawn with permission from Butler, D. L., Grood, E. S., Noyes, F. R., and Zernicke, R. F. Biomechanics of ligaments and tendons.** *Exerc. Sport Sci. Rev.,* **6, 125–82, 1978.**

stiffer. Since less elongation accompanies the increase in force, the fibres deform less.

Another physical factor that can influence the tendon's response to tensile force is its length. Longer fibres mean greater elongation at the same load (Fig. 1.9). Thus, the ideal situation is to have long fibres and plenty of them.

Because a tendon's mechanical behaviour depends on its physical size, force elongation curves must be adjusted to remove the effects of these physical parameters before comparisons can be made between tissue from different tendons. Dividing the force by the cross-sectional area yields the force per unit area, known as stress; dividing the change in length by the original length determines the relative amount of elongation, known as strain, that has occurred. The result is the familiar stress-strain curve (Fig. 1.10), which is similar in appearance to the load elongation curve (Fig. 1.9) but is independent of physical dimensions.

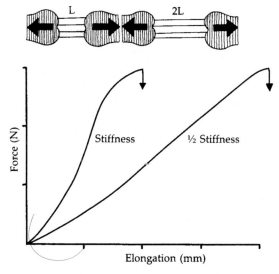

With longer fibres:
↑ Elongation to failure
↓ Stiffness
  Strength is the same

**Fig. 1.9 Effect of length on tendon behaviour. The longer tendon is stretched less at the same load application; thus less physical deformation takes place. Redrawn with permission from Butler, D. L., Grood, E. S., Noyes, F. R., and Zernicke, R. F. Biomechanics of ligaments and tendons.** *Exerc. Sport Sci. Rev.,* **6, 125–82, 1978.**

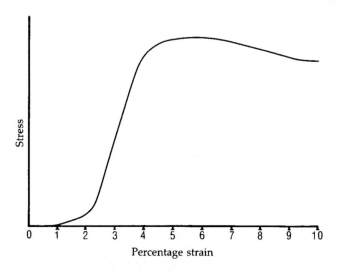

**Fig. 1.10 Stress–strain curve for the tendon.**

## Time

All connective tissues, including tendon, are viscoelastic; that is they exhibit both fluid and solid properties. Thus the mechanical behaviour of tendon is rate dependent as well as size dependent. For example, the rate at which force is applied plays an important role in the amount of force that the tendon can withstand. The rate of the tendon's lengthening is usually referred to as the strain rate, or the rate of deformation. Characteristically tendons and ligaments can withstand larger forces when the forces are applied rapidly.

Another time dependent feature of connective tissue is relaxation. If a tissue is stretched rapidly until a certain level of strain is reached and then is maintained at this fixed length while the force is measured, the forces seem to decrease over time (Fig. 1.11) until an equilibrium point is reached. Conversely, if a load is applied rapidly and maintained while the length is allowed to vary, the tissue lengthens with time (Fig. 1.12).

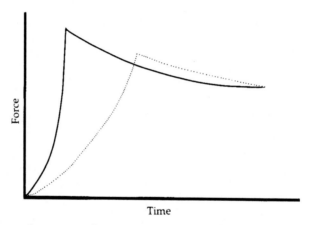

Time

**Fig. 1.11  A force–time curve demonstrating that the tension 'relaxes' (bears less load) after elongation to a fixed length.**

When a soft tissue specimen is deformed at a constant rate and then allowed to return to its original length at the same rate, while the force is monitored, there is a difference in the two curves; that is, less force is borne at the same length. This represents a loss of energy during the loading process, usually in the form of heat. This phenomenon is called hysteresis (Fig. 1.13).

The properties of relaxation, crimp, and hysteresis are all features of viscoelastic materials. Although it is not essential to know them by name, the principles illustrated are very important in understanding concepts presented later in this book. A simple example will illustrate the points just mentioned. If, in stretching the hamstring muscle group, we apply a stretch (tensile force)

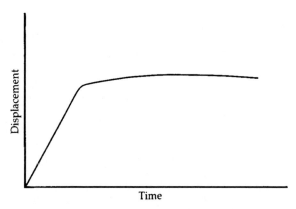

**Fig. 1.12  A length–time curve showing that the tendon lengthens with time at a constant load, a phenomenon called creep.**

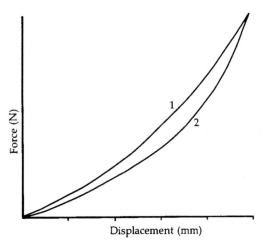

**Fig. 1.13  The difference between the slopes of the two curves shown here represents a loss of energy during the loading process. This is known as hysteresis.**

and maintain it, then the soft tissue will elongate with time because of the property of relaxation. Also, some heat will be released. This may partially explain why gentle stretching exercises can be used to warm up muscles.

## Metabolic activity

For many years tendon was mistakenly assumed to be metabolically inert except in growing animals. It is true that tendon is much less active than more cellular tissues such as muscle or liver. Gerber *et al.* (1960) measured the rates of turnover of rat collagen in various tissues, and found that of tendon collagen to be 50 to 100 days as compared with 50 days for muscle and 30 days for liver. If we compared these rates to those of actively growing tissue (for example, one to two days in the uterus during pregnancy), then the rate does seem slow. Growth of collagen involves a balance between two processes: synthesis and degradation. During growth, or following injury, synthesis exceeds breakdown and the total amount of collagen increases. When growth ceases, the two are balanced. As we age, the mechanical properties of our tendons change. These changes may be partly responsible for the increased incidence of tendinitis in older people. An age related decrease is seen in the crimp angle, thus decreasing the toe region in the tendons stress–strain curve (Fig. 1.7). Water content, collagen turnover, and the number of fibroblasts within the tendon, all decrease with age. Landi *et al.* (1980 *a,b,c*), found, in rabbits, that enzymes of both the anaerobic and oxidative pathways decreased with age with oxidative activity ceasing at maturity. They interpreted this as indicating a decreased potential for biosynthesis, or repair. Interestingly, levels of these enzymes increased following injury, and decreased as healing took place. As a result of these changes, tendon becomes stiffer with age, more susceptible to injury, and less able to repair itself. Tendon may also suffer from pathologic degenerative changes which are considered further in the etiology of tendinitis in Chapter 2.

A number of factors can affect the metabolism of collagen: altered genetic expression, hormones, nutrition, nervous control, drugs, exercise, and so on. Genetic factors may govern the number of cells in a given tissue and the amount of protein produced by these cells. Many connective tissue disorders are genetically determined. Hormones such as corticosteroids, inhibit the production of new collagen and promote the removal of already formed collagen. Insulin, testosterone, and estrogen however have the opposite effect. Vitamin C is vital for collagen synthesis. Deficiency in this vitamin causes failure in protein production by fibroblasts and may even induce their reversal to more immature cell types. Similarly, decreased levels of Vitamin A and of many B vitamins result in decreased collagen synthesis.

Since proteins are composed of amino acids, an adequate supply of these via dietary protein is necessary. Carbohydrates are also important in forming the gel-like matrix surrounding the collagen fibrils (ground substance, p. 5).

The role of nervous activity in the control of protein synthesis remains unclear. Muscle and tendon atrophy, and their collagen content decreases when their nerve supply is interrupted. However, these changes also occur during immobilization and may be at least partly due to mechanical causes. Inactivity results in increased collagen degradation (Vailas *et al.* 1981), decreased tensile strength (Tipton *et al.* 1975), and decreased concentration of metabolic enzymes (Vailas *et al.* 1978). Exercise, however, increases collagen synthesis, concentration of metabolic enzymes, and the size, number and tensile strength of the fibres (Booth and Gould, 1975).

As tendon is less metabolically active than muscle (i.e. less cellular), it takes longer for tendon to atrophy and hypertrophy than muscles. One of the postulated mechanisms for tendon ruptures in anabolic steroid users is that the muscles hypertrophy faster than the tendon, and thus the tendons are relatively weaker. This concept of (relatively) decreased metabolic activity helps to explain the recalcitrance of some cases of tendinitis to treatment, and will be expanded on in later sections on etiology and treatment.

Clearly, tendon and other connective tissues are metabolically active despite earlier misconceptions. Only recently has research interest in this area been renewed, because of the long held belief that the metabolic activity was so low as to be almost inappreciable, and healing slow and imperfect. Therefore, the roles of the various factors mentioned here remain to be determined.

# 2 Etiology of tendinitis

## The mechanics of tendon injury

Tendon is remarkably strong: its tensile strength is 49–98 N mm$^{-2}$ (Elliott 1965). Most values for force and stress in the literature are given in kilograms or kilograms per square millimetre; however the correct units are in newtons (N) or pascals (Pa). Thus the value we cite from Elliott (1965) is more properly stated in units of stress or 49–98 mega pascals(MPa). Throughout this book we used the correct units which means that most values cited have been converted from their original ones. There is a large gap between the stress that causes tendon failure and physiologic loads. The latter are reported to produce less than 4% strain (Elliott 1965). This is the 'safe' zone of the stress-strain curve (see Fig. 1.7) and it represents the straightening of the crimped collagen fibres when tendon is perfectly elastic and recovers its original length after the load is removed. Using muscles from rabbit hind legs, Elliott (1965) found that tendons of fusiform muscles transmit a maximum tension no greater than 25 MPa, whereas those of pennate muscles transmit less than 15 MPa (Fig. 2.1). Both he and Walker *et al.* (1964) suggested that tendon is probably never stressed to more than one quarter of its ultimate tensile strength during normal activities.

The muscle force may be replaced by two perpendicular vectors (represented by arrows in Fig. 2.1), with one oriented in the tendon's long axis. The size of each vector is determined by the angle of orientation of the muscle fibres. The lateral components largely cancel each other out, if both parts of pennate muscle are equally active, leaving a tensile force to be applied to the tendon in series with the muscle. Pennate muscles, therefore, exert less tensile force on the tendon because of the greater angle between the longitudinal axis of the muscle and the tendon. This is true even though muscle fibres of fusiform and pennate muscles are capable of producing equal amounts of force (Alexander and Vernon 1975).

There are few studies in which the tensile forces have been estimated at the time of injury. Zernicke *et al.* (1977) estimated a force of approximately 17 times the body weight acting on the patellar tendon of a skilled weightlifter at the moment of tendon rupture. For a 71 kilogram man whose tendon is

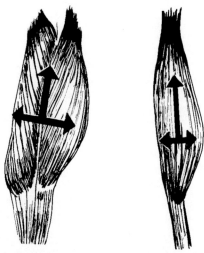

**Fig. 2.1  The force produced by a muscle can be resolved into two vectors, one in the long axis of the muscle or limb and the other perpendicular to it. The lateral vector is really the sum of the two vectors as shown here. Pennate muscles have obliquely oriented fibres, which means that more of their force is laterally directed than that of fusiform muscles (right). Since these vectors cancel, the vertical force on the tendon is seen to be less for pennate muscles, as noted by Elliott (1965) and Alexander (1974).**

assumed to have a cross sectional area of 200 mm$^2$ (2 cm$^2$) the stress on the tendon would be 29.6 MPa. This load is certainly larger than a quarter of the value cited by Elliott (1965). Indeed, during kicking, forces of up to 5200 N (26 MPa) have been estimated (Wahrenberg *et al.* 1978), leaving these authors to suggest that forces, if repeated, may damage the patellar tendon. Given an adequate time following such stresses, the tendon can recover but reapplying force before this recovery has taken place, may lead to injury.

Most tests of tendon tensile strength are performed under non physiologic conditions by using isolated tendon specimens and subjecting them to purely tensile loading. Tendons are rarely stressed like this *in vivo*. Barfred (1971) studied the anatomy, physiology, and mechanics of the bone/muscle/tendon group in general. Tendon was most vulnerable when:

- tension is applied quickly;
- tension is applied obliquely;
- the tendon is tense before the trauma;
- the attached muscle is maximally innervated;
- the muscle group is stretched by exterior stimuli; or
- the tendon is weak in comparison with the muscle.

These situations occur commonly in athletics where maximal effort is made, movement is uncertain or unexpected, or gravity or an opposing muscle stretches a contracting muscle. The variety of circumstances that can occur during sports means that while much valuable information can be gained from experimental studies, the extrapolation of results to the athletic environment remains largely hypothetical. Elliott (1965) mentions that in cases of injury, one should look for an alteration in the normally straight angle between the bone of insertion and the muscle belly. This may lead to an unequal distribution of stress in parts of the tendon that would then form the most likely sites of rupture. An example is the twisting of the Achilles tendon during its course through the leg to insert on the calcaneus (see Chapter 4).

## Pathology: what happens to the tendon?

Tendon in the resting state has a wavy configuration that appears as regular bands across the surface of the tendon (Fig. 1.4). When the tendon is stretched, the wave pattern disappears. The disappearance of the wave pattern means that the collagen fibres have been straightened. Provided that the tendon has not been stretched by more than 4%, it will immediately resume its normal appearance if the force is released.

If larger loads are applied and the tendon is elongated by more than 4%, then the collagen fibres themselves are subjected to stress. This corresponds to region II of the stress-strain curve (Fig. 1.7). The size and number of the collagen fibrils will determine the amount of force that can be applied before damage occurs. At 4–8% strain, the collagen fibrils slide past one another; at 8–10% strain, the tendon begins to fail and resists less force. First, some of the cross-links between neighbouring molecules break (Fig. 2.2). Because of tendon's uniaxial composite structure, the force is shared and individual fibres are less likely to be overloaded (as long as they are linked to their neighbours). As more and more cross-links are broken, the weakest fibres rupture and the tendon loses its composite structure. This increases the load on the remaining

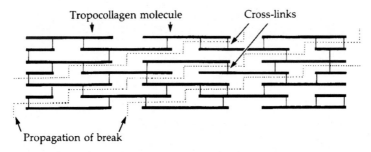

**Fig. 2.2 Tropocollagen molecules are held together by intramolecular and intermolecular bonds or cross-links. As these bonds break, the process spreads through the remaining tendon molecules.**

fibres. Continued application of force results in sequential fibre failure and, ultimately, rupture of the tendon.

Since even the largest physiologic loads fall within the limit of 12% strain, the changes that occur during tendinitis probably take place primarily at the molecular level and so are not visible to the eye. In addition, the sliding of the fibrils and the interposed matrix may cause a shearing force that can damage the tendon microvasculature. The reduction in vascular supply is important since this is the vehicle by which oxygen and other nutrients reach the interior of the tendon. Oxygen is especially important as it is essential in establishing the cross-links between the tropocollagen molecules.

Thus, the injured tendon is one with microscopic or macroscopic damage to both its structural units and its blood supply. In this state the tendon is predisposed to further injury, since time is required for healing to take place. This healing begins with the inflammatory response and is usually accompanied by pain, the first clinical sign of tendinitis. If the tendon is not given time to respond to injury and subjected to continued stress, degenerative changes occur which further weaken the tendon and become a source for chronic symptoms.

## Tendon healing

Tendon, like other soft tissues, heals in stages. An understanding of these stages is important since the physical and chemical environment during each stage affects the healing process. Most studies of connective tissue healing have been carried out on incisional wounds where the tendon or skin has been completely divided. These are not the best models for healing in clinical tendinitis, where damage is usually microscopic. Nevertheless, the principles remain the same, with the difference lying only in the degree of response.

All musculoskeletal tissues, including bone, follow the same broad pathway to healing after acute injury. The three stages of this pathway are: inflammation, repair, and remodelling. Chronically injured tendons have a somewhat different histological picture and are discussed later in the chapter.

### Inflammatory response

The damage to the tendon microvasculature that occurs at the time of injury, results in bleeding and increased permeability of the remaining intact vessels, so that fluid accumulates in the area (if the area is large, this is readily seen as swelling around the tendon). The rupture of damaged cells releases chemicals that initiate this increase in vessel permeability (vasodilatation) and that act as signals to other cells to come to the area to aid in cleaning up the damaged tissue. Some of the chemicals released help break down the connective tissue elements.

The inflammatory response begins when the injury occurs and may last from 2–7 days. Although it may seem destructive rather than reparative, it is necessary to draw cells involved with the healing process to the area, such as white blood cells. Eliminating the inflammatory response by drug adminis-tration can delay or interrupt healing.

Although the inflammatory response is necessary to initiate healing, it should only last a short time. Hypoxia results from impaired circulation caused by stasis of the extracellular fluid, and the acidic environment in the area of injury causes an increase in proteolytic activity, which may be detri-mental to the surrounding healthy connective tissue if the inflammation is prolonged.

## Repair

Overlapping with the inflammatory phase, the repair phase may start as early as 48 hours after the injury and last from 6 to 8 weeks. Ground substance pro-liferation predominates early in the repair phase (until day 3 to 4). The ground substance is the gel-like matrix that surrounds the collagen fibrils and is composed of proteins, carbohydrates, and water. The ground substance is produced by the fibroblasts that are found in the surrounding connective tissue. The existence of an adequate amount of ground substance is necessary for the aggregation of collagenous proteins (which also are produced by the fibroblasts) into the shape of fibrils. Until day 5 following the injury, a high proportion of the collagen is soluble, or immature, because cross-links have not yet formed between the tropocollagen molecules. Soluble collagen is much more susceptible to breakdown by enzymes that the inflammatory response activates (hence the importance of limiting the inflammation after the initial phase of injury). From day 6 to day 14, the proportion of insoluble collagen increases as cross-links form between the tropocollagen molecules. The rate of collagen degradation concomitantly decreases, since cross-linked collagen resists enzymatic degradation. Around day 12 to 14, the initial colla-gen laid down (Type III) is replaced by Type I collagen, which is more stable as it promotes increased cross-linking between molecules than Type III.

## Remodelling

From day 14 onwards (up to one year), collagen continues to increase and begins to organize into fibrils that are laid down randomly. Tension now begins to play an important role in the healing process because the collagen fibres reorient themselves in line with the tensile force applied to the tissue. In fact, the rate of collagen fibre formation is directly related to the functional state of the affected area. The amount of tension that is necessary, or optimal, remains unclear. All tendons are subjected to some tension through contraction of their attached muscles, but the amount may be markedly reduced if joint motion is prevented. Stress on the collagen fibres also produces a piezo-electric effect, resulting in the development of an electric potential. Since collagen molecules have an electric charge, this may affect their alignment as well, and may be a means by which tension helps reorient the collagen fibrils. The use of electric stimulation to enhance tendon healing, in a manner similar to techniques now used to promote fracture healing, is just beginning to receive attention.

Unfortunately, however, the remodelled scar tissue will never have strength equal to that of the premorbid tendon. The final construct may be up to 30% weaker biomechanically than normal, healthy tendon. Patients are never told they can be 'normal' or 'good as new', but that they may have a tendon to withstand all normal stresses, a very 'functional' tendon.

## Chronic injury

In cases of chronic tendon complaints, there is usually an element of degenerative change in the tendon itself—tendinosis. The inflammatory phase is markedly diminished, thought to be due to hypoxia and age related changes. Focal areas of overload and/or hypovascularity have a decreased cell stress-response capability, which initiates the degenerative process. Dystrophic calcification (seen in both the Achilles and patellar tendons), fibrinoid degeneration, cartilage metaplasia, and angiofibroblastic hyperplasia (chronic granulation tissues seen in tennis elbow) are all potential sequelae. For symptomatic control, the inflammation must be limited and the tendon then strengthened gradually to meet the demands placed on it (remodelling). Needless to say, a tendon with degeneration and damaged vascularity will take longer to heal than one injured acutely and statements made to patients should reflect this fact.

## Forms of treatment

The variation in classification and in location of tendinitis, together with the lack of agreement as to etiology in many cases (or even exact location), has led to a bewildering assortment of treatment techniques. Most are based on scientific principles, but are not equally well adapted to different patients. For example, a retired man with tennis elbow may respond more readily to the suggestion of rest as a form of therapy than a young volleyball player with jumper's knee who is in the middle of the season. These factors must be considered when a form of treatment is chosen, since patient compliance is the single largest factor determining the success or failure of treatment.

Treatment can be divided, broadly, into rest and activity. However, because many forms of treatment combine both rest and activity, this classification has been modified and is presented in Table 2.1.

**Table 2.1 Forms of treatment for tendinitis.**

| Treatment | Used in this stage of healing |
| --- | --- |
| Rest | 1, 2, 3 |
| Stop activity | |
| Cast immobilization | |
| Taping/support | 1, 2, 3, 4 |
| Physical modalities | 1, 2, 3 |
| Ice | |
| Electric stimulation | |
| 'Deep heat' | |
| Ultrasound | |
| Drugs | 1, 2, 3 |
| Anti-inflammatories (oral) | |
| Steroids (injection) | |
| Exercise | 3, 4 |
| Stretching | |
| Strengthening | |
| Surgery | 1 (rupture) or 4 (chronic) |

Rest

Rest may mean anything from briefly stopping any pain causing activity to having the affected limb placed in a cast for 3 to 6 weeks. In general, if an activity causes pain of such magnitude that one cannot perform the activity, then it is wise to stop that activity *for a short time*. This is only common sense and appears even more logical if we consider that pain is a clinical sign of the inflammatory reaction of tissue and thus acts as a warning signal.

Equally, if a person ceases permanently to participate in an activity that produces pain or discomfort, then it is likely that he or she will no longer suffer that discomfort. This is unacceptable to most athletes and economically impossible for a patient whose tendinitis is related to their occupation.

Cast immobilization for long periods is unnecessary and undesirable from both a physiologic and mechanical point of view. During joint immobilization tendons lose from 20–40% of their ground substance (Akeson *et al.* 1967), and new connective tissues formed during periods of immobility may contain less elastin. Furthermore, the removal of mechanical influences on the newly formed collagen means that orientation of the collagen fibrils cannot take place, and they are laid down randomly, which reduces the tensile strength of the healing tendon. Those fibres not subjected to tension are resorbed in the remodelling process, which continues until the tissues collagen content returns to normal. For this reason, inactivity is to be discouraged after day 14 (before day 14, movement may disrupt healing rather than promote it) following the injury, since it is detrimental to collagen fibre orientation and to tendon strength, which depends on the number, size, and orientation of the fibres. In addition to the effects on the injured tendon itself, immobilization has profound effects on muscles and other soft tissues in the immobilized limb. Muscle wasting and weakness, joint stiffness, and lack of proprioception occur in other areas besides those injured. Thus, after cast removal, a great deal of rehabilitation may be necessary to return an athlete to competition.

For these reasons, we do not advocate cast immobilization of injured tendons. If rest is necessary, withdrawal from the sport may be advised for one to two days (longer if necessary). Alternatively, limited rest may be achieved through the use of taping, elastic supports, or braces (Fig. 2.3). The concept of limited rest means that the injured tendon is used, but is protected from stress which may damage it further, with the patients using pain as their guide to activities. The use of measures such as those of Fig. 2.3, should *always* be augmented by a program designed to correct the initial cause of the tendinitis.

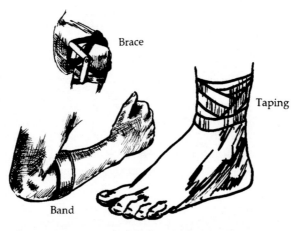

Brace

Taping

Band

**Fig. 2.3 Some devices may assist the athlete by restricting motion to a non-painful range.**

## Drugs

### Non-steroidal

The inflammatory reaction in initiating healing and the desirability of limiting this reaction, if it is prolonged beyond its normal time limits (2 to 7 days) are important. This period is the same as that advised for rest in cases of acute tendinitis.

The prescription of any drug is, of course, made by the physician. There are a variety of types and brand names. The individual physician prescribes what is considered to be most suitable.

Aspirin is a potent anti-inflammatory drug and is available without prescription. Its use is convenient in cases where pain is not intense or symptoms fluctuate. Nonetheless, the patient should obtain advice on dosage from a professional before self-administering any drug.

The consensus seems to be that anti-inflammatories should be limited to use in the acute phase of an injury and for a short period of time only. Longer term use may retard healing and lead to gastrointestinal problems. A short trial (10 to 14 days) may be indicated in chronic cases that have an associated inflammatory component to break the inflammatory cycle.

### Corticosteroids

Steroids are also anti-inflammatory drugs and injections of these drugs are used in the treatment of tendinitis. There are numerous reports in the literature, however, of tendon ruptures following steroid injection. Experimental studies have shown that the tensile strength of the tendon is decreased following steroid injection and the production of collagen and ground substance is reduced (Wrenn et al. 1954; Kennedy and Baxter-Willis 1976). Degenerative changes occur in both the tendon and the peritenon, and the physical presence of the drug causes circulatory stasis which is detrimental to the tendon's microvasculature. Corticosteroid injection is especially contraindicated in the middle third of the tendon (where the blood supply may be wholly dependent on vessels from the peritenon), and in cases where continued physical activity is expected (or suspected), since this will increase the risk of rupture. The latter instance would involve any athletic activities and even normal walking for cases of Achilles tendinitis and jumper's knee.

If corticosteroid injection is employed, it should be placed into the tendon sheath only and followed by ice application to decrease the inflammatory reaction at the injection site. Physical activity should be reduced for two to three weeks. Since such injections frequently improve symptoms dramatically on a temporary basis, it is unlikely that the patient will refrain from activity, and the athlete may return to training, competition, or work prematurely. Although some authors have failed to find any deleterious effects associated with steroid injection, the overwhelming majority are of the opposite opinion and discourage the use of steroids in treating tendinitis. In light of the biochemical and mechanical effects, all of which are negative, the authors support this view.

## Physical modalities

Physiotherapists treat tendinitis with such physical measures as ultrasound, short wave diathermy or other forms of 'deep heat', electrical stimulation, massage, heat, cold, and whirlpool.

*Cold*: decreases inflammation by reducing the rate of chemical activity and vasoconstriction caused by brief periods of ice application (5–15 minutes). This should decrease swelling in the area, as a result of increased permeability of the dilated capillaries. Cold is also an effective analgesic, decreasing sensory nerve conduction for 30 minutes to 2 hours after application. The safest and most effective method of applying cold therapy is by means of crushed ice and a damp towel; however immersion in ice water is also very effective. There are also numerous other means of applying cold therapy. Ice should be applied for a limited time (less than 15 minutes) and repeated every one to two hours in acute cases. For cases of chronic tendinitis, ice should be applied after any activity that produces discomfort.

*Ultrasound* therapy: uses high frequency sound waves to produce a mechanical effect on newly formed scar tissue. The piezoelectric effect is again at work, but this time in the opposite direction (i.e. an electric signal received by the sound head causes a crystal to vibrate, producing mechanical waves). The application of these waves renders the tissue more susceptible to subsequent remodelling by appropriate tensile forces, thus ultrasound should be followed by exercise. Ultrasound can also have a heating effect, and is believed by many physiotherapists to reduce inflammation. This latter claim, however, has no real scientific basis since it has not been proven experimentally. Ultrasound has been shown by some to increase tensile strength and energy absorbtion capacity of the tendons, interpreted as accelerating healing.

*Deep heat*: is a term that refers to any means by which heat is concentrated at a tissue level below the skin surface. It has the same effect as local heat application (increased temperature and blood flow). It may also reduce the stiffness of the connective tissue, making it a useful preliminary to stretching exercises.

*Electric stimulation*—transcutaneous neurologic stimulation (TNS or TENS): is becoming more and more commonplace. Simply, it replaces the pain signal with a new one—an electric current. The pain relief lasts for varying lengths of time depending on the severity of the symptoms. Since this treatment (as currently used) affects only the symptoms of tendinitis, other measures must be taken to eliminate the cause of the problem. One potentially interesting application of electric stimulation has already been alluded to—that of improving healing. Electric stimulation of healing fractures has become an accepted form of therapy, and electric stimulation of muscles to increase strength, is commonly used also. At the Nova Scotia Sport Medicine Clinic, electric stimulation has been applied to healing surgically repaired dog anterior cruciate ligaments; these stimulated ligaments have a greater tensile strength than the controls. Enwemeka (1989 *a,b*) has shown that electrical stimu-lation enhances protein synthesis and increased tensile strength of healing tendons, and as such may be useful for rehabilitation. However, at the moment it seems that the additional collagen produced is purposeless collagen unless it is aligned along the lines of stress through movement and use of the extremity creating tension across it.

*Massage*: is another popular physiotherapeutic maneuver to treat tendinitis. It refers to a technique called *deep friction*, which is used to break down scar tissue. It is very uncomfortable but effective when properly done by a skilled therapist.

*Surgery*: in patients whose tendinitis has been resistant to other forms of treatment, surgery may be necessary. The usual reason is to remove the build up of scar tissue that accompanies repeated trauma and to encourage revascularization. The scar tissue usually forms as a result of increased collagen synthesis in response to injury, but is immature and disorganized so that it adds little to the strength of the tendon. The removal of scar is followed by suturing of the tendon or leaving it to heal in a lengthened state (as in many cases of tennis elbow). Some formal post surgical immobilization is usually required.

Although surgical intervention is unquestionably necessary following spontaneous tendon rupture, its value in cases of chronic tendinitis is less certain. Because surgery is usually followed by immobilization, an extended period of rest and rehabilitation exercises, it is difficult to ascertain to what the clinical improvement is actually attributable. Surgery may be indicated in rare instances in which non surgical measures failed to effect any improvement in the patient's symptoms. The role of surgery could be better evaluated if controlled clinical trials were performed in which different groups of patients with the same diagnosed disorder received different forms of therapy, surgery included. This would allow a direct comparison of methods: however it is seldom done.

*Exercise*: Tension, and therefore activity, are important in the orientation of newly forming collagen fibrils. Increase in the size and mass of bone and muscle with activity, and their wasting with inactivity, have been recognized for many years. Indeed, most rehabilitation programs are devoted to reversing the weakness and atrophy that follow injury or immobilization.

More recently investigators have observed the same effects of use and disuse on ligaments and tendons. Noyes *et al*. (1974) studied the mechanical properties of anterior cruciate ligaments of monkeys after 8 weeks of cast immobilization and found a 39% decrease in maximum failure load and decreased stiffness. Even after 20 weeks of post immobilization reconditioning, the ligament had only partially recovered. In the same study, localized exercise was shown to be of no benefit in preventing weakening of the ligament during cast immobilization, leading these authors to suggest that localized exercise could not reproduce and simulate the total force placed on an extremity in a normal ambulatory state. Swine trained for 12 months showed increases in stiffness, ultimate load, and total weight of extensor tendons (Woo *et al*. 1975); and Barfred (1971) noted that wild rats had much stronger ligaments than domesticated rats. Numerous other studies on rats (Tipton *et al*. 1967; Zuckerman and Stull 1973) and dogs (Tipton *et al*. 1970) show the same results—activity strengthens ligaments and tendons, inactivity weakens them. More recent studies have reaffirmed this fact.

Woo *et al*. (1975) showed that repeated exercise increases both the mechanical properties (material composition) and the structural properties (hypertrophy) of the tendon. A number of mechanisms have been implicated in the changing of connective tissue properties:

- changes in the synthesis and degradation equilibrium of collagen;
- changes in collagen cross-links on an intermolecular and intramolecular level;
- alterations in water and electrolyte content of connective tissues;
- changes in arrangement, number, and thickness of collagen fibres (Noyes *et al*. 1974).

Mechanical stresses on the connective tissue must be necessary, since rats in a swimming training program do not show the same increase in ligament strength as those placed on a treadmill running program (A.C. Valais personal communication).

One drawback of the experimental results just described is that they were all from studies involving animals. It is difficult, if not impossible, at present to perform similar experiments on humans since they are reluctant to volunteer to have large ligament or tendon specimens removed! The development of miniaturized strain gauge techniques may make feasible the *in vivo* testing of human tendon, an area in which much research is needed but which remains virtually unexplored.

*Laser stimulation*: as a modality, this has a reasonable track record on improving skin wound healing, however its effect on tendon healing is less clear. As with electrical stimulation, it may improve the amount of collagen in the tendon, but exercise and tension placed across the tendon is necessary to orient this collagen along the lines of stress and make the tendon stronger. This seemed to be confirmed by Reddy *et al.* (1998) who found that a combination of laser therapy and electrical stimulation increased the biochemical properties of tendon (i.e. more collagen was produced), but they were unable to show a statistically significant increase in the strength of the tendon.

## Summary

The application of force to the tendon via muscle contraction produces tensile stress in the attached tendon. The amount of stress is related to the magnitude of the force generated by the muscle, the direction of the force application, and the physical dimensions of the tendon. The most likely etiology for tendinitis is disruption of the tendon's structural integrity by tensile stresses that exceed the strength limits of some of the smaller fibrils or fibres. On a large scale this may result in actual tendon rupture.

   Tendon healing proceeds through three stages. The first stage (inflammation) brings the needed cells for repair to the area and eliminates necrotic material. During the second stage (repair), new collagen is produced. A variety of physical modalities and rest are used to control the clinical symptoms (primarily pain) during this period. Next is the remodelling stage, in which tissue remodelling occurs. During this stage, which lasts until the collagen content and tendon structure are near normal, tensile stress should be introduced to optimize healing, since tension appears to play an important part in directing the organization of the new tissue. The role of exercise in the form of tensile stress for treatment of soft tissue disorders is firmly supported experimentally by animal studies. The results of such studies form a theoretical basis for the exercise program that forms the cornerstone of the therapeutic program at the Nova Scotia Sport Medicine Clinic. The rest of this book is devoted to the description of this program and its application to various tendon disorders.

# 3 Exercise and the muscle-tendon unit

Having presented the ground work for understanding tendon structure, behaviour under normal and abnormal circumstances, and methods of healing, we will now consider the relationship between exercise and the tendon.

Muscles become stronger if they are exercised; if muscles are stretched, they become longer. But more than muscle, however, responds to exercise. Because of the functional integrity of muscle-tendon units, exercise also affects the tendons. Yet for many years this fact was ignored, owing to the continuing belief that tendons were mere inert bands of connective tissue.

The recent interest in tendons (and ligaments) has stimulated investigations into the effects of exercise on these structures.

## Type of exercise

The basis for movement and exercise is muscle contraction. Characteristically we tend to regard contraction as a shortening of the muscle that occurs as the thick (myosin) and thin (actin) filaments slide past one another. Yet during many activities the overall muscle length does not change, and in some cases it may actually lengthen. These differences in muscle behaviour during activity have led to the classification of muscle contraction (or exercise) as concentric, eccentric, or isometric (Fig. 3.1).

### Isometric

When the shoulder muscles contract to counter the downward forces produced by carrying an object, the muscles are acting isometrically. Of course, no contraction is truly isometric, since some shortening *must* occur at the muscle fibre level. However, no change in the overall length of the muscle takes place. As a result, this type of contraction is referred to as *static*.

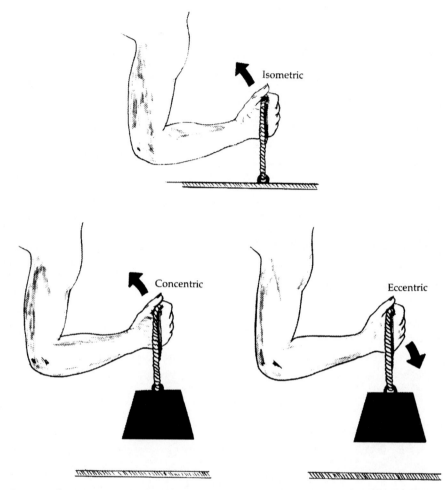

**Fig. 3.1 Three types of exercise: no movement occurs (isometric), the weight
is lifted (concentric), the weight is lowered (eccentric).**

## Concentric

During concentric contraction, muscles shorten while producing tension.
Lifting weights against gravity makes use of this type of movement. In effect,
the internal force generated by the muscles overcomes the force of the
external resistance.

## Eccentric

This kind of contraction is the opposite of a concentric one. When muscles
contract eccentrically, they lengthen while producing force. The external

resistance in this case is greater than the internal force produced by the muscles. Eccentric contractions are very common, since every movement in the direction of gravity is controlled by them, including sitting, descending stairs, and lowering weights. Also, most movements are preceded by a preliminary countermovement in the opposite direction; when direction is changed, eccentric contraction is usually involved.


## Work and energy


All muscle contractions require energy to perform work. In order to produce energy, fuel must be consumed. Muscles generate mechanical energy, or work, by using the chemical energy (fuel) produced from food. The processes of fuel transformation can proceed either with oxygen (aerobically) or without oxygen (anaerobically). Although these methods are very different, they both produce ATP (adenosine triphosphate), the chemical substance that allows muscles to contract. Eventually chemical energy becomes mechanical energy.

Mechanical work is the effect of applying a force to an object (be it a weight, a limb, or the body itself) and causing it to move. In the terms of a physicist or engineer, mechanical work is the product of force and distance. Muscles can perform two types of mechanical work: *positive* and *negative*.

Muscles accomplish positive work when they shorten and overcome an external resistance such as gravity. The potential energy of the system on which the muscles act increases and the object being acted on moves in the same direction as the muscle contraction. Lifting a weight is a simple example of this type of work.

Negative work involves displacement of an object in an opposite (negative) direction to the force exerted by the muscles. In other words, movement is in the same direction as the external force. The muscles lengthen, and the potential energy of the system decreases. Lowering the weight just lifted is an example of negative work.

Potential energy is the energy due to gravity, and so it is the product of an object's weight (mass multiplied by acceleration due to gravity) and its height relative to the ground or some other suitable reference point. This is recognizable as nearly identical to the earlier definition of mechanical work. In positive work, when a muscle contracts to lift a weight, it produces more force than the force due to gravity acting on the object. As the object's distance from the ground increases, so does its potential energy. In negative work, the muscle force is less than the force due to gravity (weight) and the potential energy decreases. These concepts are illustrated in Fig. 3.2.

Positive work accelerates the body or limb. Negative work decelerates a

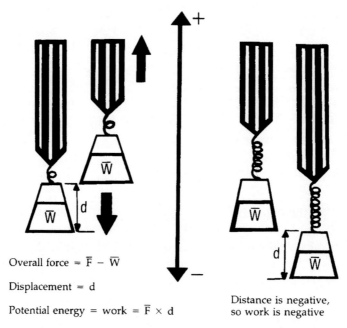

Overall force = $\bar{F} - \bar{W}$

Displacement = d

Potential energy = work = $\bar{F} \times d$

Distance is negative,
so work is negative

**Fig. 3.2 Potential energy increases with positive work and decreases with negative work.**

moving object. In most cases, the terms *positive* and *negative* may be considered synonymous with concentric and eccentric contraction respectively.

## Force–velocity relationship

The force produced by skeletal muscle is dependent on both the speed of shortening and the length of the muscle at any instant in time. A typical curve of the relationship between velocity of muscle contraction and the force produced by the muscle is represented by Fig. 3.3. This curve is similar for isolated muscle fibres, muscles involved in simple tasks such as elbow flexion (Wilkie 1950), or large muscle groups involved in more complex movements such as running or jumping.

The relationship between muscle force and speed of shortening differs for eccentric and concentric contraction. Figure 3.3 illustrates that in eccentric exercise, the force increases as the velocity of contraction increases (at least to a certain point). In contrast, during concentric exercises the force decreases as the speed of contraction increases.

The force–velocity relationship may have important applications to training. To increase muscle force under conditions of negative work (eccentric contraction), the limbs should be moved as rapidly as possible. During

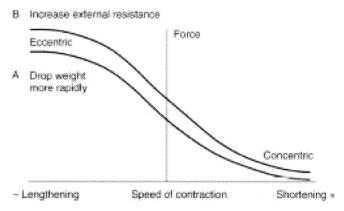

Fig. 3.3 The force–velocity relationship for muscle (general case) showing that tension is higher during lengthening contractions and increases with speed of lengthening.

concentric exercise, movement should be performed slowly to maximize force production. Figure 3.3 shows that the force production during eccentric contraction appears to be greater than during concentric exercise. Since this force is transmitted by the tendon to its insertion, the tendon is subjected to larger loads during eccentric exercise.

## Force–time relationship

To move efficiently, coordination between the signals for muscle contraction and force production is necessary. In sport, the minimization of time lags between these two is extremely important. There is a latent period of approximately 55 milliseconds (Wood 1977) between the signal for muscle contraction (from the brain) and the onset of muscle electrical activity (as seen on Electromyography or EMG) and a further delay between the appearance of EMG activity and tension in the muscle. Thus the second delay is referred to as the *electrical mechanical delay* (EMD) (Komi and Cavanaugh 1977). These authors have shown that EMD is shorter under conditions of eccentric contraction, suggesting that this is a strategy for producing the greatest force in the least time.

## Force–length relationship

When the joint between two adjusted bones changes its angle, so does the mechanical action of the muscle. This is a function of two variables: the length of the muscle and its distance from the joint centre of rotation (Fig. 3.4).

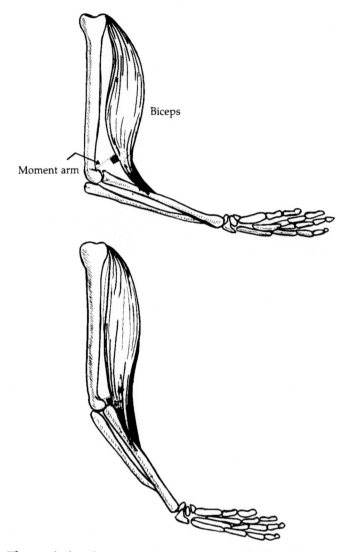

**Fig. 3.4 The variation in moment arm (perpendicular distance between muscle and joint) and muscle length with elbow movement. Note that muscle length increases during extension, but the moment arm becomes much smaller. At 90°, however, the moment arm reaches a peak length. It is at this angle that the largest torque is produced.**

As muscles contract, they produce rotation at joints because the line of action of the muscle is located at a distance from the joint's centre of rotation. This distance is referred to as the *lever*, or *moment*, arm of the muscle. It is a line perpendicular to the muscle's line of action extending from that line to the joint's centre of rotation. The mathematical product of the force produced by the muscle and its moment arm is known as the *joint moment*, or *joint torque*. During most human motion analysis, it is only this variable that can be estimated. The amount of force produced by muscles increases as the length of the muscle increases (up to a certain point). This increases the joint torque. The joint moment also increases if the distance between the muscle and the joint centre of rotation increases. Thus, joint movement alters both the length and the moment arm of the muscle and thereby controls the joint moment. There is an optimum joint angle at which the product of force and moment arm is largest. As the joint moves away from this position, less torque is produced either because the muscle is too short or too long, and thus produces less force, or because the moment arm has become shorter. Most maximum joint torques occur at mid-range. For example, the maximum joint torque at the elbow occurs at approximately 90° flexion. The relationship between joint angle and muscle force is shown in Fig. 3.5.

For isolated muscle fibres, the force production increases with length until a critical length is reached, then decreases because less filament overlap is possible. This relationship also holds for whole muscles but is complicated by

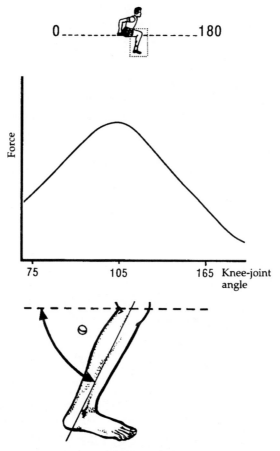

**Fig. 3.5 Variation in force as knee extends, because the moment arm decreases and the muscle shortens after midrange.**

alterations in the moment arm. Thus, the relationship between joint angle and force production is not simply the relationship between force and length, but involves change in the mechanical action that the muscle is able to exert on the joint.

## Neurologic influences

Muscle contraction and force production are governed not only by mechanical factors such as length and lever arm, but also by the activity of the muscle. The basic component of the neuromuscular system is the motor unit—an anterior horn cell, its motor axon, and all the muscle fibres it innervates. There are varying numbers of motor units within the muscles. Muscle contraction can be graded by increasing either the number of motor units that are active at any particular time or the frequency of their firing. Differences in firing frequency have led to the designation of two motor unit types: slow twitch (ST) and fast twitch (FT). The latter are able to produce more force because they have higher firing frequencies and larger muscle fibres, or more fibres per motor unit.

Muscle contraction is under both voluntary and reflex control. The muscle length and the force and speed of the contraction are monitored by sensory receptors in the muscle and tendon—the muscle spindles and the Golgi tendon organs (GTO). The former provide feedback to the central nervous system concerning muscle length and velocity, while the GTO, located in the tendon near the musculotendinous junction, provides information about the force acting on the tendon. The signals from these two receptor types have opposite reflex effects on the muscles (Fig. 3.6). The muscle spindles signal tends to

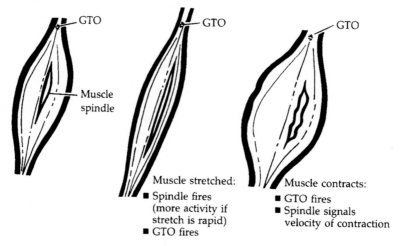

Fig. 3.6 Two types of muscle-tendon receptors and how they are affected.

produce muscle shortening (since the spindles are stretched by elongation of the muscle, being parallel with it). The GTO is affected most by active muscle contraction and produces reflex relaxation of the muscle. The actions of the different receptors allow the muscle to respond to both passive and active lengthening or shortening, and alter the sensitivity of the muscle, possibly allowing it to produce more force at certain positions.

The preceding paragraphs describe neurologic control of the muscle-tendon unit in its simplest form and are included to illustrate the complex interaction that allows muscle force production to be modified. The reader is referred to other sources such as texts of neurophysiology for a more complete description.

## Muscle elasticity

The muscle-tendon unit, despite its complexity, can be modelled as a two-component system: a contractile component (CC) in series with an elastic component (SEC) (Komi 1979). This model is represented in Fig. 3.7a.

It is the rearrangement and length of the contractile and elastic muscle-tendon components that produce force in all three types of muscle contractions. In isometric contraction, force is generated by the contractile component and is accompanied by stretching of the series elastic component. In concentric contraction, some stretching of the SEC occurs, but most of the force is produced by the actual sliding of the muscle fibre filaments past one another. During eccentric contraction, the muscle is lengthening as it contracts, which

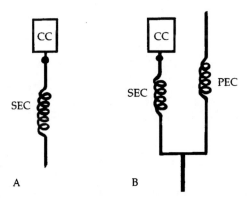

**Fig. 3.7 Theoretical models for muscle behaviour. A. The simplest, with just a contractile component (CC) and series elastic component (SEC). B. Slightly more complicated because a parallel elastic component (PEC) is shown in parallel with both the CC and SEC. This represents connective tissue such as muscle sheaths.**

stretches the SEC and allows it to contribute to force production. The presence of the series elastic component may account for the high tension that occurs in eccentric contraction (Fig. 3.8). The total force generated is the sum of that produced by the contraction of the CC and by stretching of the SEC.

The actual location of the SEC is a matter of some controversy. Although most authors agree that the tendon, because it is in series with the muscle, must perform at least part of the SEC function, many believe that the major portion of the SEC resides in the myosin cross-bridges, that are stretched during that part of muscle contraction when the actin and myosin are in contact and moving away from each other. Other connective tissue elements in parallel with the muscle may also contribute to force production at lengths far above the resting length. This is the parallel elastic component (PEC), illustrated in Fig. 3.7b. The PEC is thought to play only a minor role in most physiologic activities (Thys *et al.* 1972).

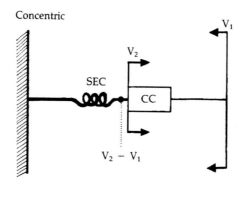

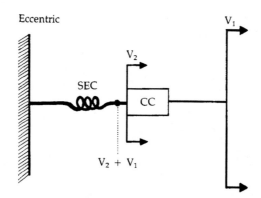

**Fig. 3.8 In concentric contraction, the velocity and force are contributed to by the CC only, since the muscle ends are moving to 'unload' the SEC. The opposite is true in eccentric contractions—the SEC is stretched and contributes to force production. Redrawn with permission from Komi, P. V. Neuromuscular performance: factors influencing force and speed production.** *Scand. J. Sports Sci.*, **1, 2–15, 1979.**

In most movements, muscle action seldom begins from a static starting position. The push-off phase in running is preceded by the heel strike and foot-flat phases. Similarly, a downward motion of the body with knee flexion, almost always precedes the upward jumping motion in volleyball and basketball (in other words, an eccentric contraction of the quadriceps) (Fig. 3.9).

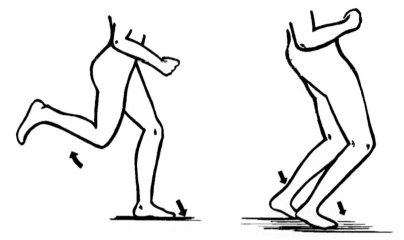

**Fig. 3.9 Eccentric contractions are required in both running and jumping.**

Thus, in most sports, muscle is stretched before it contracts concentrically. This mechanism enhances muscle force production by stretching the SEC and allowing it to contribute. Reflex activity (via muscle spindles and GTOs) may also contribute to force production by increasing the stiffness of the muscle by making it 'springier'. Many researchers have shown that eccentric contraction enhances muscle force production and is less costly metabolically than concentric contraction (Bosco and Komi 1979; Cavagna *et al.* 1965, 1968; Komi 1973, 1979; Komi and Bosco 1978; Thys *et al.* 1972).

More force is produced at less metabolic expense as the body improves the efficiency of muscle contraction by using the stored elastic energy of the SEC.

## Eccentric exercise program

The above is the scientific background for the 'eccentric exercise program' used at the Nova Scotia Sports Medicine Clinic to treat tendinitis. After careful questioning of many afflicted athletes, we began to realize that eccentric contraction was somehow involved in the production of tendinitis. In the case of a basketball player, for example, we discovered that the exact moment of greatest pain occurred in landing from a jump, although pain often would be felt during take-off as well. Further testing revealed that in many cases pain could be reproduced in the clinic only by eccentric loading. If we refer to what we know about muscle-tendon mechanics, this seems logical. Greater force production during eccentric contraction translates into greater stress in the tendon during this type of activity.

Noting this relationship, a training program was developed to (theoretically) strengthen the actual tendon tissue. We reasoned that the forces to which the tendon was subjected during activity were causing damage to the tendon microstructure at the collagen fibre level. Although various types of weight training program were frequently part of the athletes existing training program, the emphasis was usually on concentric or isokinetic exercises. We added eccentric exercises designed to reinforce the muscle-tendon unit and focus the training regime on three functional areas: length, broad, and speed of contraction.

*Length*: Stretching would be an integral part of the program. By increasing the resting length of the muscle-tendon unit, we could lessen the strain (deformation) taking place during the same range of joint movement. Research has indicated that stretching may strengthen the tendon or make it more resistant to strain and increase the range of motion of the relevant joint. Wiemann and Hahn (1997) found that while both warming up and stretching (static and ballistic) increased joint range of motion, only warm-up did so by reducing the resting tension of muscle.

They proposed warm-up and stretch work through different mechanisms should be used to increase flexibility, which is the key to reducing muscle-tendon injury, and thus we use both in the eccentric program to maximize their effects. The role of warm-up in the prevention of muscle (and hence tendon) injury has been well documented (Safran *et al.* 1988; Strickler *et al.* 1990).

*Load*: Increasing the load would clearly subject the tendon to greater stress and would form the bases for the progression of the program. This principle of progressive overloading forms the basis of all physical training programs. Since eccentric exercise produces the highest levels of force in the tendon, it would seem to be the most efficient way of stimulating it to hypertrophy. There is support for the concept that the effects of training are specific (Friden *et al.* 1983; Stafford and Grana 1984; Stanton and Purdam 1989; Kellis and Baltzopoulos 1995), therefore eccentric exercise should be used to increase eccentric muscle-tendon strength, which has been shown to decrease eccentric overload injury (Schwane and Armstrong 1983).

*Speed of contraction*: The force on the tendon is related to the speed of muscle contraction (see Fig. 3.9). Increasing the speed of the movement would also increase the load on the tendon and increase the specificity of the program so it better simulates the mechanism of injury, which usually occurs at relatively high velocities.

Based on these factors, the following eccentric exercise program has been developed:

1. Warm-up and stretch
   (a) General warm-up
   (b) Static stretch
   (c) Hold 15–30 seconds
   (d) Repeat 3 to 5 times.
2. Eccentric exercise
   (a) Three sets of ten repetitions
   (b) Progression:  Days 1 and 2—slow
                            Days 3 to 5—moderate
                            Days 6 and 7—fast
   (c) Increase external resistance; after day 7, repeat cycle.
3. Stretch, as prior to exercise.
4. Ice: crushed ice or ice massage applied to tender or painful area for 5–10 minutes.

## Pain

The presenting symptom of tendinitis is pain; indeed, that is why the athlete seeks help. Pain, which indicates ongoing inflammation of the tendon, is the most common measure used to classify the degree of tendinitis severity. We devised the following system of symptom classification, similar to that used by other authors (Fox *et al*. 1975; Perugia *et al*. 1976):

Level 1—no pain
Level 2—pain only after extreme exertion
Level 3—pain with extreme exertion and for 1–2 hours afterward
Level 4—pain during and after vigorous activities
Level 5—pain during activity that forces termination
Level 6—pain during daily activities

Table 3.1 shows the effect of pain on athletic performance. Although pain is a subjective assessment, this classification of tendinitis severity can be a criterion for evaluation. We use the degree of reported pain, included in both the pre- and post-exercise assessment, to determine the efficacy of the exercise program as a means of assessing the rate of progression of the program.

The intensity of the exercise should be such that pain, or discomfort, is experienced in the last set of 10 repetitions. This discomfort indicates that a

**Table 3.1  Classification system for the effect of pain on athletic performance.**

| Level | Description of pain | Level of sports performance |
|---|---|---|
| 1 | No pain | Normal |
| 2 | Pain only with extreme exertion | Normal |
| 3 | Pain with extreme exertion and 1 to 2 hours afterward | Normal or slightly decreased |
| 4 | Pain during and after any vigorous activities | Somewhat decreased |
| 5 | Pain during activity and forcing termination | Markedly decreased |
| 6 | Pain during daily activities | Unable to perform |

slight overloading of the tendon is occurring, which is necessary to increase its strength. We have observed that no pain indicates insufficient loading, and so no improvement in symptoms occurs. However, extreme pain, especially throughout the entire 30 repetitions, is a sign that too much force is being applied. This may act to worsen the patient's condition. Incorrect evaluation of the level of pain or discomfort is the major cause of program failure.

As the strength of the connective tissue increases, the pain will decrease and the force on the tendon can be increased until the pain recurs. This force increase is achieved by gradually increasing the speed of contraction from days 1 to 7.

In our experience patients generally follow the progression outlined in Fig. 3.10.

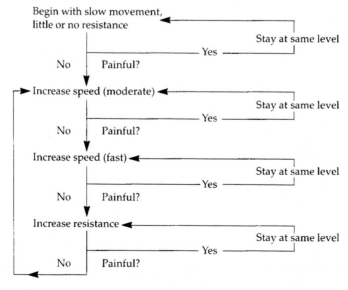

**Fig. 3.10  General outline of eccentric exercise program.**

## Controlling inflammation

Microstructural damage to the collagen fibres and disruption of the tendon microvasculature results in inflammation, which is heralded by pain. We have already discussed the deleterious effects of inflammation on the tendon (Chapter 2) and the importance of controlling the inflammatory response. The application of ice immediately after trauma, minimizes chemical activity and reduces pain. For these reasons, ice should be applied at the end of each treatment session and at more frequent intervals during treatment of acute tendinitis. Other measures, such as drugs or physical modalities, are left to the discretion of the individual physician or therapist. We have rarely found them necessary.

## Avoidance of activity

Tendons need mechanical stress to hypertrophy, and as such, activity should be encouraged early *with pain used as a warning signal to limit the duration and intensity* of such activity. Nikolaou *et al.* (1987) and Taylor *et al.* (1993) have both shown that contractility of the muscle-tendon unit is not lost despite severe muscle injury, and that the muscle-tendon unit should have enough strength to undergo early functional rehabilitation. These two studies deal with muscle injuries, which are obviously at a different point in the musculo-tendinous unit, so extrapolation of these results to chronic tendon injuries should be done very judiciously; it has been our clinical experience however, that most chronic tendon injuries are capable of early functional rehabilitation (provided the pain level is monitored closely). Early controlled activities should be a treatment goal in all cases, with brief periods of rest reserved for severely painful cases. Prolonged rest has no role in our treatment program.

## Summary

This chapter has considered the different types of muscle contraction and the effects of each in terms of force production. Although there is opacity of experimental data dealing with the behaviour of muscle during lengthening contractions as compared with the volume that exists concerning shortening contractions, results indicate that force increases with length for both eccentric and concentric contractions. The relationship between force and velocity differs: force increasing with the velocity of muscle contraction during eccentric exercise but decreasing as the velocity increases during concentric exercise. The literature also suggests that eccentric contraction is a means by which muscles may maximize their force production while minimizing time delays and energy expenditure. Using this information and our clinical experience, an exercise program to treat tendinitis was developed at the Nova Scotia Sport Medicine Clinic. Pain, the cardinal sign of tendinitis, is used as both a classification of severity and a yardstick of treatment progress.

# 4    Achilles tendinitis

All running athletes, including anyone who participates in the sport that involves running and jumping, risk Achilles tendinitis occurring. Older athletes seem to be at a higher risk, in part due to age and vascularity related degenerative changes. Since the fitness explosion and the development of jogging into a common recreational pastime and keep fit method, more people have been exposed to the risk of Achilles tendinitis than ever before. In fact, Achilles tendinitis has become by far the most common athletic injury (Clancy 1982).

Like other tendinitidies, Achilles tendinitis is difficult to treat, proving frustrating for both patient and therapist. This frustration has bred a plethora of treatment regimes, all of which meet with varying success at resolving the tendinitis.

The mechanics of Achilles tendinitis, the structure of the Achilles tendon and some of the treatment regimes are renewed here. We also adapt the eccentric exercise program outlined in Chapter 3 to this specific athletic injury problem.

## Structure of the Achilles tendon

The Achilles tendon is the common tendon of the gastrocnemius and soleus muscles. These two muscles are often referred to as the calf muscles, or triceps surae. The gastrocnemius arises from the lateral and medial femoral condyles, to which it is connected by strong, flat tendons. The soleus originates from the posterior surfaces of the tibia and fibula, and lies beneath the gastrocnemius (Fig. 4.1). The individual tendons of the gastrocnemius and soleus combine distally to form the Achilles tendon. Because of this arrangement, the Achilles tendon receives muscle fibre attachment from the soleus until just a few centimetres above its insertion onto the calcaneus. Note that the soleus and gastrocnemius contribute separately to the formation of the Achilles tendon, and this contribution varies among individuals. The gastrocnemius portion varies from 11–26 cm in length. In comparison, the soleus contribution varies from 3–11 cm.

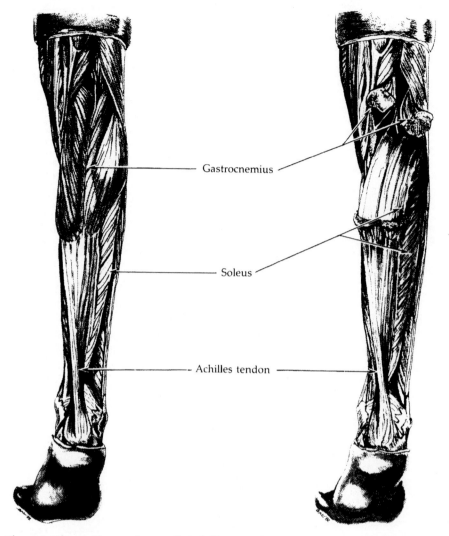

**Fig. 4.1 The calf muscles and Achilles tendon. Note the insertion of the soleus into the tendon until quite far down and the twist as it descends.**

The Achilles tendon, initially fan-shaped and somewhat flattened near the gastrocnemius, becomes more rounded as it approaches the calcaneus, where it expands slightly to attach to its posterior surface. As it expands, the tendon gradually converts to fibrocartilage and stiffens as a result. Barfred (1971) postulates that this stiffness protects the tendon from oblique traction, just as the stiff cuff fitted on a flex close to an electric iron, prevents buckling of the flex.

A second feature of note is that the tendon twists as it descends. The gastrocnemius portion usually makes up the more lateral and posterior portion of the tendon. As a whole, the tendon appears to rotate laterally as it descends.

This rotation begins approximately 12–15 cm above the insertion and where the soleus begins to contribute fibres to the tendon. The degree of rotation depends on the amount of fusion between the gastrocnemius and soleus portion of the tendon. These two muscles may be separate through nearly the entire length or fused, depending on the individual. Minimal rotation seems to be associated with lengthy fusion.

Cummins *et al.* (1946), examined one hundred tendons and described three patterns of rotation:

- Type 1: the gastrocnemius contributes two thirds of the posterior part of the tendon and the soleus contributes one third;
- Type 2: the gastrocnemius and soleus each contribute one half; and
- Type 3: the soleus makes up two thirds of the posterior part of the tendon and the gastronemius makes up the other one third.

Type 1 is most common (52%), followed by Type 2 (35%), and Type 3 (13%).

This twisting produces areas of stress concentration in the tendon, caused by a 'sawing' action of one part of the tendon on the other (Barfred 1971). This concept of spiralling of the fibres of the Achilles tendon has led some authors to conclude that it plays a part in the genesis of the so-called 'watershed area' of hypovascularity 2–6 cm above the tendon's insertion (Galloway *et al.* 1992). This is analogous to wringing out a dishtowel. The clinical observation that the watershed area is the most common site of injury (including rupture), dovetails nicely with the theory that injury occurs when stresses exceed the body's reparative capacity. This reparative capacity would obviously be decreased at an area of decreased blood supply to the tendon.

The insertion of the Achilles tendon into the calcaneus is protected by two synovial bursae—the subcutaneous bursa, between the skin and the tendon and the retrocalcaneal bursa, between the tendon and the upper part of the calcaneus (Fig. 4.2). Inflammation of either of these bursae (bursitis) may mimic the signs and symptoms of Achilles tendinitis. Like other tendons, the Achilles tendon is composed of the familiar fibres, primary fibre bundles, and fascicules. The tendon is surrounded by a fine sheath called the epitenon. This sheath continues into the interior of the tendon, as the endotenon, to surround the primary and secondary fibre bundles (fascicles). The endotenon contains the internal vasculature of the tendon derived mainly from a bed of vessels in the mesotendon, lying just beneath the tendon. This bed of vessels is an anastomosis from larger blood vessels in the area.

Covering the epitenon is a filmy layer of areolar tissue, the paratenon, which contains blood vessels running in a circular pattern around the epitenon. It acts as an elastic sleeve, allowing the tendon to move freely against, yet in continuity with, the surrounding tissue. The epitenon and paratenon together are often referred to as the *peritendon* (Fig. 4.3).

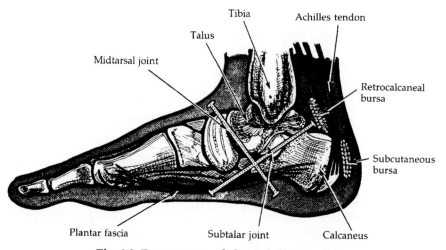

**Fig. 4.2  Bursae around the Achilles tendon.**

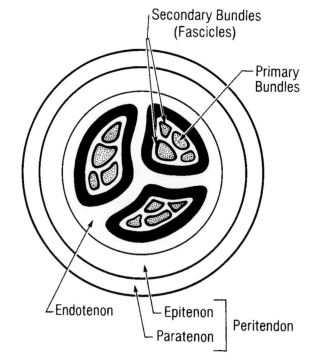

**Fig. 4.3  Layers of sheaths surrounding the Achilles tendon.**

## Vascular supply

The Achilles tendon receives its blood supply at three locations: the musculo-tendinous junction, the tendon/bone junction, and along its length. The blood supply derived along the length of the tendon from the underlying mesotendon is most important. Small blood vessels arise from the branches of the posterior tibial and peroneal arteries, and anastomose in the mesotendon. From there they assume a course parallel with the longitudinal axis of the tendon in the endotendon.

## Classification of Achilles tendon disease

It is difficult to classify Achilles tendon disorders because of the possibilities of different types. For example, many authors distinguish between a 'true' tendinitis and tenosynovitis. The term *tenosynovitis*, however, does not strictly apply in the case of the Achilles tendon, since it is covered by a peritendon, not a synovial sheath. Recognizing this, many authors now prefer the term *peritendinitis* or *paratenonitis*. They propose a classification of tendinosis and peritendinitis, with the former indicating disruption of the actual tendon and the latter being inflammation of the tendon sheath. This definition can extend also to combinations of tendinosis and peritendinitis, as well as partial rupture.

Undoubtedly there are cases in which symptoms are due to inflammation of the tendon sheath, that is, peritendinitis. But the number of these cases that do *not* involve injury to the tendon as well must be very small. Since the injury may be at the microscopic level, subsequent inflammation can take place without visible change in the tendon. Sometimes symptoms can be precipitated through pressure on the tendon, such as from a high heel counter on a running shoe or a tightly laced skate, and cause irritation of the peritendon alone. More commonly, either the retrocalcaneal or subcutaneous bursa is involved.

Most symptomatic cases of Achilles tendinitis involve trauma to the actual Achilles tendon, as described in Chapter 2. The injury may be on a fibrillar level or greater. The resulting inflammatory response causes pain, which increases with the magnitude of the injury. As a result, we prefer to use the classification system outlined in Table 3.1. Injuries that cannot be classified by this system are usually easy to diagnose since they are caused by an external force, such as a blow or pressure from footwear. Although not initially considered 'true' tendinitis, the inflammatory changes accompanying these injuries may cause weakening of the tendon and predispose it to tendinitis.

## Etiology

## Mechanics

Tendons are adapted to withstand tensile forces and their fibres are aligned in response to this type of force. In areas where tendons must withstand or 'absorb' large forces, they are usually found to be long in relation to their accompanying muscles because the tendon is much stronger than the muscle per unit area. Long tendons are also able to 'store' some of this force for brief periods and use it to perform movement, much as a stretched elastic band assists movement when it is released (Murray *et al.* 1978). (This is the concept of elastic energy discussed in Chapter 3.)

At first glance, the Achilles tendon seems well suited to withstand the external forces encountered in walking and running, since generally its fibres are longitudinally oriented. However, recall that the tendon twists as it descends, producing areas of stress concentration and ringing out the vascularity as one part of the tendon saws across another. This saw-like action is compounded by the fact that the tendon is not homogenous but receives interdigitating fibres from the soleus.

The ankle is a hinged joint with motion in one plane only (sagittal) which leads to the assumption that any force applied to the Achilles tendon produces motion only about an axis through the ankle joint. This apparent simplicity is contradictated when we consider that motion at the subtalar joint also affects (and is affected by) the Achilles tendon. Motion at the subtalar joint occurs in the frontal and transverse planes, producing inversion/eversion and abduction/adduction movements, respectively. Movement in the transverse plane twists and untwists the Achilles tendon. Inversion and eversion place unequal tensile forces on different parts of the tendon which can result in a bow string effect in the Achilles tendon (Smart *et al.* 1980).

Barfred (1971) emphasizes the fact that all tendons passing one or more joints with axes of movement at right angles to each other, may be exposed to oblique traction. He notes that a 30° change in position of the hindfoot results in one side of the tendon being elongated 10% more than fibres on the other side. However, these movements are necessary to allow accommodation of the foot to uneven ground.

Various authors (Alexander and Vernon 1975; Ljungqvist 1968; Smith 1975) have estimated the force in the Achilles tendon during such activities as walking, running, and landing from a jump. These forces range from approximately 1962–2354 N in walking, to 3924–5886 N in running, and up to 8729 N in fast running. The stress on the tendon (force per unit area) can be calculated by dividing these values by the tendon's cross-sectional area. The maximum value of stress for the mammalian tendon is estimated to be 49–98 MPa (Elliott 1965). Table 4.1 shows the stresses on the Achilles tendon during various activities, based on a theoretical cross-sectional area of 75 $mm^2$.

**Table 4.1  Stress in Achilles tendon with different activities.**

| Activity | Area ($mm^2$) | Force (N) | Stress (MPa) |
|---|---|---|---|
| Walking | 75 | 1962–2354 | 26.1–31.4 |
| Running, slow | 75 | 3924–5886 | 52.3–78.5 |
| Running, fast | 75 | 8729 | 117.7 |
| Jumping | 75 | 1962 | 26.1 |

Stresses applied to the Achilles tendon during athletic activities, however, appear to exceed these maximum levels. Unfortunately, the most accurate information available on tendon behaviour during activities such as walking and running comes from animal studies, where forces and strains can be measured directly. Data on human tendons have been derived from laboratory studies or estimated from film and force platform data. It is difficult to make direct comparisons between stresses estimated during activities and those determined under laboratory conditions, because the latter are derived from tests performed on isolated tendon specimens that are elongated at a constant rate until failure. Under these controlled conditions, the strain rates may be considerably lower than those that take place during sporting activities, which alters the load that the tendon is able to bear (Kear and Smith 1975; Lochner *et al.* 1980). Thus the maximum tendon stress value of 49–98 MPa may be lower than that which occurs at higher strain rates, and may be lower than the actual maximum strength of the tendon. The imposition of factors such as heel varus or valgus, tibial torsion, or excessive tightness in the calf muscles, may also lead to areas of stress concentration in the tendon, increasing the likelihood of microtears (Fig. 4.4).

## Role of eccentric contraction

Ljungqvist (1968), in a review of 92 cases of partial Achilles tendon rupture, lists the following situations as most likely to cause injury to the Achilles tendon:

1. Pushing off with the weight bearing foot while simultaneously extending the knee, common in sprinting or running uphill. The calf muscles are maximally contracted.
2. Sudden and unexpected dorsiflexion of the ankle, such as slipping on a

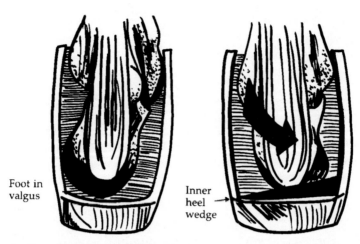

Foot in valgus

Inner heel wedge →

**Fig. 4.4  A valgus hindfoot stretches the inner part of the tendon more. This is readily corrected with a small median heel wedge.**

stair or stumbling into a hole, where the heel drops suddenly. The calf muscles are moderately contracted but become maximally contracted in reflex to the sudden stretch.

3. Violent dorsiflexion while the foot is plantar flexed, such as in jumping and falling. The calf muscles are maximally contracted, and sudden movement leads to marked stretching of the muscle and particularly the tendon.

All these examples involve eccentric contraction of the muscle, that is the muscle is contracting and lengthening as the tendon is stretched. Athletes suffering from Achilles tendinitis characteristically feel more pain during an eccentric movement and can frequently recall specific motions, much like those mentioned, that are painful.

There appears to be a contradiction between the fact that isolated tendon specimens are stronger when tested at higher strain rates and the clinical impression that sudden movement appears more likely to injure the tendon. On the basis of experimental findings, one would expect the tendon to increase its resistance to injury as it is stretched more rapidly. This cannot be readily explained except that extremely rapid movements do not allow time for protective measures, such as relaxing the muscle, to occur. The stresses on the tendon with differing strain rates have not been investigated experimentally, nor are the normally occurring strain rates known. Thus, more research is needed before the exact nature of the interaction between rates of loading and strain can be understood.

## Footwear

Footwear may contribute to Achilles tendinitis in a number of ways. Loose heel counters and narrow heels may not afford sufficient stability to the subtalar joint. Clement *et al.* (1984) make a very convincing case that abnormal biomechanics, mainly over pronation of the foot, contribute to the avascularity of the watershed area. The reader is referred to their article for a more detailed explanation.

In addition a high, poorly padded heel counter may cause undue pressure on the tendon, leading to subcutaneous Achilles bursitis or retrocalcaneal bursitis.

Inadequate heel elevation may also be a factor. Flat shoes may cause the tendon to be stretched farther at heel strike. Since most walking shoes have heels, switching to flat shoes may overstretch the shortened tendon. This effect suggests that athletes who use flat shoes (such as tennis players or basketball players) may be particularly vulnerable to Achilles tendinitis, yet runners are more likely to suffer it because of the many more times that the tendon is loaded—each time the foot strikes the ground.

To lessen the propensity for Achilles tendinitis, the shoe sole should be flexible and soft enough to cushion heel impact during running. A rigid sole increases the distance from the ankle at which the force must be applied during push-off (moment arm), thus increasing the ankle joint moment. This moment is 'balanced' by one in the opposite direction created by the force of the calf muscles acting through the Achilles tendon. The mathematical product of this force and the perpendicular distance (moment arm) between the tendon and the ankle joint centre equals the magnitude of this moment. Thus, as the joint moment increases, so does the force in the tendon. Shoes should be examined to ensure that they bend readily in the forefoot at a level corresponding to the metatarsophalangeal joints.

## Training

Sudden alterations in style or quantity of training can produce microtrauma in the Achilles tendon. Certain changes are particularly likely to precipitate tendinitis:

- changing shoes;
- adding hills or sprints to regular training;
- running on uneven ground;
- changing running surface (as when ground freezes);

- inadequate emphasis on warm-up and flexibility;
- beginning another sport such as basketball, tennis, or squash;
- sudden increase in mileage;
- resumption of training after a long period of inactivity;
- single severe competitive or training session (triathlon, marathon, etc.).

## Examination

### Case history

The importance of the case history cannot be over-emphasized. Since pain is the usual symptom that causes the athlete to seek help, the examiner must determine where the pain is, when it occurs, how long it lasts, and the time elapsed since symptoms were first noted. The duration of pain and its severity are particularly important in classifying the degree of tendinitis. Questions concerning other causative factors, such as training changes, should be included in the initial work-up. This will help to reveal whether any training factors are implicated in causing the tendinitis. Careful examination of the running shoe and the foot, in both standing and non weight bearing situations, is mandatory for physicians and trainers attempting to isolate a cause for the presenting tendinitis. This will enable the examiner to see whether structural or alignment problems are contributing to the problem.

### Clinical examination

The injured tendon should be palpated along its length in both the relaxed (plantar flexed) and taut (dorsi flexed) positions and compared with the contralateral side. This is best done with the patient lying prone. Swelling of the peritenon, unlike thickening of the tendon tissue, is superficial and feels less 'solid'. Pressure on the swollen segment often produces pain. Not infrequently, a thickened area will be noted. This may indicate a previous injury to the tendon or areas of focal degeneration.

Examination of joint range and muscle tightness should also be performed. Make the athlete lean forward against a support, with the heel on the floor and the knee straight. Ask the patient to bend the knee of the extended leg. The bent knee should allow more dorsi flexion because the gastrocnemious is partially relaxed. If dorsi flexion does not increase, then tightness of the soleus muscle is present.

Functional tests, such as hopping on one foot or dropping the heel rapidly over the edge of a step, may be used to determine whether eccentric contraction of the calf muscles is involved in the injury. These tests frequently produce pain on landing during hopping or pain at the end of the range of movement in dropping over a support, and are important in a complete assessment of the problem.

## Other possible disorders confused with Achilles tendinitis

Achilles tendinitis may be confused with other athletic injuries, including some of the following:

1. Bone bruises: (a) caused by a direct blow to the calcaneus, usually at the plantar surface; (b) relieved by removing pressure on the painful area.
2. Bursitis: (a) either retrocalcaneal or subcutaneous; (b) usually related to external pressure from shoe or skate; (c) some cases are due to internal pressure from posterosuperior calcaneus especially during dorsi flexion.
3. Plantar fasciitis: (a) inflammation of the calcaneal attachment of plantar fascia; (b) characterized by tenderness at the point of insertion and sharp pain during weight bearing activities, especially during push-off; (c) etiology is varied, may be weak foot intrinsic muscles, overweight, flat foot, and so on; (d) symptomatic relief most easily obtained with orthotics; (e) physiotherapy or anti-inflammatory drugs may be useful.
4. Fracture: (a) a stress fracture may result from repetitive trauma or from the same factors that cause tendinitis; (b) pain increases with intensity and is felt at rest; (c) activity is usually impossible.
5. Muscle tear: (a) usually related to a single traumatic episode; (b) accompanied by swelling, bruising, and pain.
6. Posterior tibial tendinitis (shin splints): (a) pain along the medial border of tibia; (b) causes much the same as for Achilles tendinitis; (c) often faulty foot alignment is involved, best solved with the use of orthotics.
7. Compartment syndrome: (a) pain in lower leg related to increased pressure in one of fascial compartments of the leg; (b) requires careful evaluation and possible surgery.

## Treatment

Conservative treatment (as outlined in Chapter 2) is generally used to deal with Achilles tendinitis. Modalities include rest, anti-inflammatory drugs, ultrasound, orthotics, and cast immobilization. When these methods fail, as they frequently do, surgery may be performed. Although these treatments may relieve symptoms, recurrence is common because the basic cause of the problem is not being dealt with—an Achilles tendon too weak to do what is demanded of it. There is sufficient current (and some past) evidence to show that inactivity actually weakens the tendon structure. Thus, while rest or surgery (which is inevitably followed by rest) may succeed in relieving symptoms in some cases, these are not the treatments of choice. A vicious cycle begins, with rest weakening the tendon so that symptoms recur as soon as activity is resumed. Eventually, any rigorous physical activity provokes symptoms. Only in cases of acute tendinitis, where pain is so intense as to prevent athletic participation, should complete rest be enforced and then only until the acute symptoms subside. Anti-inflammatory drugs may be helpful during this period. Topical anti-inflammatory gels are relatively new and have been shown to be effective versus placebo (Russell 1991). This may be a better way of delivering medication to the inflamed area rather than risking potential gastrointestiral problems with the oral route.

The use of corticosteroid injections in treating Achilles tendinitis is strongly discouraged. Kennedy and Baxter-Willis (1976) have shown that physiologic doses of steroid placed directly into the normal tendon, weaken it significantly for up to 14 days after injection. The incidence of tendon rupture after steroid injection is also very high (Ljungqvist 1968).

Heel lifts have been advocated to decrease the stress on the Achilles tendon; however, some studies have questioned their merit. Reinschmidt and Nigg (1995) found that an increase in heel height did not decrease the plantar flexion moment at the ankle (which was assumed to equate with Achilles tendon loading), and that it actually increased the dorsi flexion moment initially. It is tempting to conclude that this reflects eccentric loading of the Achilles tendon but this has not been proven. Lowdon et al. (1984) compared the effect of heel lifts on Achilles tendinitis in a randomized prospective double-blind controlled trial and found that they made no difference. They found that the biggest correlation with the patient's outcome was the patient's duration of symptoms prior to entering the study.

## Surgery

Surgery has been advocated as a last resort when all other conservative measures fail. The rationale for surgery is that the fibrotic paratenon can be excised and degenerative foci in the tendon can be removed, thus leaving healthier tendon tissue. In instances where there is no overt tendon pathology, longitudinal tenotomies have been advocated to promote a vascular response.

Treatment success, defined as little or no pain and a return to pre-injury activity level, has been reported to be between 67% and 92%, with some suggestion that results may deteriorate after five years. A recent paper by Alfredson *et al.* (1998*a*) however, suggests that surgery may not be as important to outcome as a program of rehabilitation that includes eccentric exercises. They found equal results between two groups of patients, one treated surgically and one treated with eccentric exercises. All patients had previously failed conservative treatment. In light of the findings that recovery from surgery for Achilles tendinitis is slow, they went so far as to say that no patient should have surgery unless an eccentric exercise program has been tried first. The work of Clement *et al.* (1984) supports this concept, as they reported a 96% rate of good or excellent results with an eccentric exercise program and orthotics to control over pronation. In addition, it seems that an eccentric exercise program can produce satisfactory outcomes in 6 to 12 weeks, which is not possible with surgery.

## The eccentric exercise program

The program of exercise outlined in Chapter 3 can be applied to Achilles tendinitis also. The first step is a warm-up, followed by flexibility exercises for the calf muscles (Fig. 4.5). The warm-up may consist of any moderately vigorous activities such as sit-ups, push-ups, and so forth.

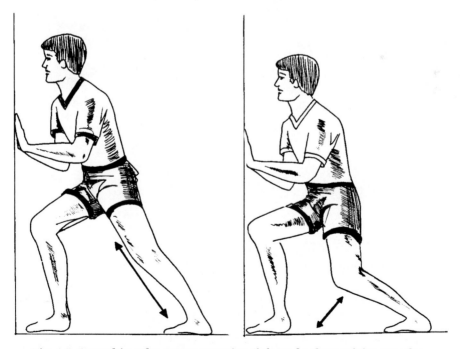

**Fig. 4.5 Stretching the gastrocnemius (*left*) and soleus (*right*) muscles.**

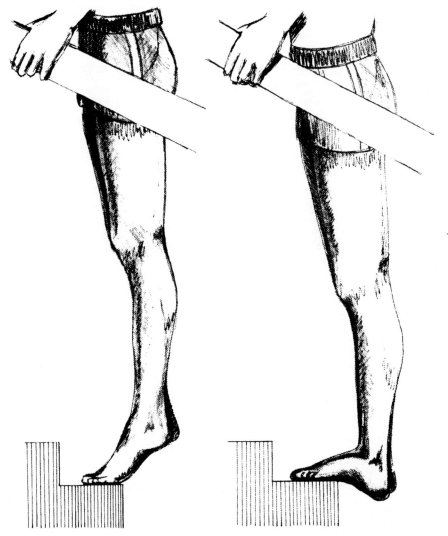

**Fig. 4.6 The eccentric exercise—drop body weight downward over the edge of support.**

Next, 3 sets of 10 repetitions of the eccentric exercises are carried out. This is most easily done by having the patient stand on the edge of a step. The body weight is supported on the ball of the foot, so the heel is free. Then allow the heel to drop downward with gravity, below the level of the step (Fig. 4.6). Progression is made by increasing the speed of movement or increasing the resistance. The program proceeds as follows: (1) weight is supported equally on both feet throughout the exercise session; (2) increase shifting of weight to symptomatic leg; (3) weight is supported on symptomatic leg only; (4) increase speed of dropping; (5) add weight to shoulders.

The severity of the initial symptoms determines the starting resistance. The indication for an increase in resistance is the absence of pain at the end of 30 repetitions. For example, an athlete whose symptoms were present during any activity, such as running on level ground, and who experienced their heel pain when dropping over the edge of the step, would start at a *slow* speed with body weight supported on *both* feet. An athlete who experiences pain only during extreme exertion, such as sprinting up hill, may start the program with weight placed on the shoulders and supported on one leg. Generally adding 10% of body weight is a suitable starting point for this phase of the program, although trial and error may change that rule. The summary of progression is shown in Table 4.2, which includes suggested starting points based on the level of symptoms.

Since each athlete varies in body weight and size, and in the severity of symptoms experienced, we recommend the program be monitored by the

**Table 4.2  Eccentric exercise program for Achilles tendinitis.**

| Week | Days | Exercise | Activity level |
|------|------|----------|----------------|
| 1 | 1 to 3 | Slow drop, bilateral weight support | Cannot participate |
|  | 3 to 5 | Moderate speed, bilateral support | |
|  | 6, 7 | Fast drop, bilateral support | |
| 2 | 1 to 3 | Slow, increased weight on symptomatic leg | Cannot participate in sports |
|  | 3 to 5 | Moderate, increased weight | |
|  | 6, 7 | Fast, increased weight | |
| 3 | 1 to 3 | Slow, weight supported on symptomatic leg | Pain during rapid drop; active in sports, but limited |
|  | 3 to 5 | Moderate, weight on one leg | |
|  | 6, 7 | Fast speed | |
| 4 | 1 to 3 | Slow, add 10% of body weight | Pain during vigorous activity |
|  | 3 to 5 | Moderate, same weight | |
|  | 6, 7 | Fast speed | |
| 5 | 1 to 3 | Slow, increase by 2.25–4.5 kg | Pain only during exertion |
|  | 3 to 5 | Moderate speed | |
|  | 6, 7 | Fast speed | |
| 6 | 1 to 3 | Slow, increase 2.25–4.5 kg | Rarely experience pain |
|  | 3 to 5 | Moderate speed | |
|  | 6, 7 | Fast speed | |

amount of discomfort the patient experiences. There should be some discomfort in the last 10 of the 30 repetitions, but pain should *not* be present throughout and the level of pain should not be extreme. Ignoring pain, the body's warning signal, means further damage may occur. Progression should not take place until discomfort is absent or minimal.

Often there will be little or no change in symptoms during the first two or three weeks of the program. Indeed, patients may experience a slight increase in the pain felt during athletic activities. This is normal but can be very discouraging to the athlete who will have to be reassured that he or she must continue the program.

The most frequently asked question during this time is, 'When will the symptoms disappear?'. This is related to the severity of the symptoms when the program began, and the prior duration of symptoms. In an athlete who experiences pain only infrequently with maximum exertion, symptoms should be alleviated within 6 weeks. Individuals with more severe symptoms, that have been present for a longer time, may only begin to see improvement in 6 weeks, and complete relief may take considerably longer.

# 5    Jumper's knee

The jumping athlete subjects the patellar tendon to tremendous forces with each explosive jumping movement. Repetition of such movements can cause trauma to the tendon, producing patellar tendinitis, or 'jumper's knee'. Basketball and volleyball players are especially vulnerable to this disorder because of the high demands placed on their quadriceps. However, athletes involved in running, cycling, kicking or other jumping events may be similarly afflicted. The incidence of patellar tendinitis has been estimated at over 40% lifetime for high level volleyball players and was seen in 15% of US military recruits in one study.

In this chapter we review the structure and mechanics of the knee extensor mechanism, the etiology and differential diagnosis of jumper's knee, and the treatment of this disorder. Again, activity in the form of eccentric exercise is stressed.

## Structure and function

The quadriceps femoris covers most of the front and sides of the femur and is the great extensor muscle of the leg. It is divided into four parts, hence its name. The rectus femoris and vastus intermedius, the most central portions of the muscle, jointly form the quadriceps tendon (Fig. 5.1). The vastus lateralis, the largest part of the quadriceps, contracts into a flat tendon attached to the lateral border of the patella and the quadriceps tendon. The vastus medialis has a broad aponeurotic attachment to the medial border of the patella and the quadriceps tendon. Its lower fibres, almost horizontally oriented, form the vastus medialis obliquus, VMO, (the characteristic bulge seen just medial to the patella when the extensor muscles are contracted). The patella lies within the quadriceps and provides protection for the knee joint. It also increases the length of the moment arm of the quadriceps, an action commonly described as 'increasing the mechanical advantage of the muscle'.

The tendons of the different portions of the quadriceps unite in the lower thigh to form a single strong tendon attached to the base of the patella. The fibres of the quadriceps tendon enclose the patella and pass over it to blend

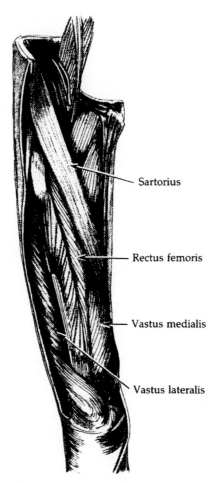

**Fig. 5.1  The quadriceps muscle (vastus intermedius not shown).**

with the ligament and patellae, or patellar tendon, which inserts on the tibial tubercle.

There is some debate as to the description of the infrapatellar portion of the quadriceps tendon. Most people consider it a continuation of the tendon of the muscle and thus call it the patellar tendon. Others claim it differs from ordinary tendons and is closer to a ligament structure. We use the term patellar tendon in our discussion.

Essentially the ultrastructure of the patellar tendon follows the description in Chapter 1. Like other tendons, it is stiffer and more avascular near its bony attachments. The reduced blood supply in these areas makes them slow to heal and prone to chronic tendinitis. Thus, we would expect the attachments to the patella and the tibial tubercle to be the most common sites of tendinitis; and, indeed, this is so.

## Sites of patellar tendinitis

There are three possible locations for patellar tendinitis (Fig. 5.2): at the insertion of on the tibial tubercle; at the inferior pole of the patellar; and at the superior pole of the patella. Interestingly, the vulnerability of these locations to tendinitis is age specific. The first is more common in growing children or adolescents, and the last in athletes over 40 years of age.

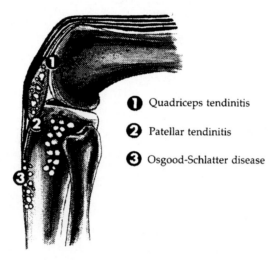

① Quadriceps tendinitis

② Patellar tendinitis

③ Osgood-Schlatter disease

**Fig. 5.2  Three common sites of patellar tendinitis (jumper's knee).**

### Insertion on tibial tubercle

In growing children, the tibial tubercle is part of the upper epiphysis of the tibia and is the 'weak link' in the extensor mechanism. The traction of the tendon on the tubercle elevates it from the tibial shaft, forming the characteristic bump of what is often referred to as Osgood-Schlatter's disease.

### Inferior pole of the patella

This is true patellar tendinitis and it occurs at the attachment of the tendon to the inferior pole of the patella. It is by far the most common site of the patellar tendinitities, and it is usually seen in individuals between late adolescence and 40 years of age. In fact, 80% of cases of patellar tendinitis in this age group are located at this site. Occasionally this type of tendinitis occurs in younger age groups and is called Sinding Larsen Johansson disease. In these cases, however, a separate area of calcification is present in the patellar tendon

(Medlar and Lyne 1978). Thus it appears very similar in etiology to Osgood-Schlatter's disease.

The etiologic factor in adult patellar tendinitis seems to be the concentration of stress that occurs at this site, owing to the narrowing of the tendon. The stress increases with knee flexion and can lead to tendinitis.

## Superior pole of the patella

This is the most common site of tendinitis in people over the age of 40. Yet, overall patellar tendinitis occurs relatively infrequently in athletes in this age group. The reason is unclear but we may speculate that the increasing stiffness of the tendon renders it more resistant to injury as the person ages. Another reason may be that we decrease demand in general on the tendon as we age, thus putting less stress across it.

The signs, symptoms, and functional disabilities are similar for all three kinds of patellar tendinitis; so is the treatment. Yet, recognition of these locations is important in differential diagnosis, as we see later in the chapter.

## The lesion

Patellar tendinitis is a chronic overload lesion in the tendon. Excessive stress in this part of the tendon during repetitive movement of the extensor mechanism of the knee results in microtearing within the tendon, followed by fraying of the tendon fibres and focal degeneration. As a useful analogy, consider a rope after some of its woven fibres have been ruptured. The ends of these fibres fray, and more stress is placed on the remaining fibres, so that they may eventually fail as well.

The lesion in the patellar tendon is usually situated in the deep fibres of the tendon near its insertion. There are two reasons for this. First, the fibres near the centre of the tendon exhibit less crimping and so are less elastic. Second, bending of the fibres with knee flexion occurs at a more acute angle near the centre of the tendon. Anatomic examination (Martens *et al.* 1982; Popp *et al.* 1997) revealed consistent findings of mucoid degeneration and fibrinoid necrosis within the tendon, thus making it a tendinosis lesion. Areas of so-called 'angiofibroblastic tendinosis' have been noted (disorganized small vessel ingrowth with disorganized collagen and tenocyte hyperplasia), as have the occasional calcific nodule. All of these dysplastic changes make up the spectrum of tendinosis. The response to injury of the tendon causes pain and weakness in the remaining fibres, predisposing the tendon to further injury, thus patellar tendinitis is usually chronic and progressive since the same loads are being applied to increasingly weaker structure. In healthy individuals, the patella is considered the weakest link in the extensor mechanism by some authors (Miskew *et al.* 1980). This means that violent quadriceps contraction on a flexed knee will cause a transverse fracture of the patella across the fulcrum of the femoral condyles. However, contractions are rarely this violent and microtrauma rather than macrotrauma occurs. This trauma will affect the tendon, if any degenerative changes are present, as it then becomes the weakest link in the system.

There are very few athletes who have not suffered some degenerative changes in their tendons owing to their sports involvement. Usually these are minor in nature, and the athlete is asymptomatic.

## Signs and symptoms

### Pain

Pain is the predominant symptom and the one that causes the athlete to seek assistance. The pain is usually very localized, so careful questioning about the exact site of pain (and having the person point out the painful spot) should be very helpful. You should note when the pain is felt, and how long it lasts since these facts indicate the severity of the injury. The role of eccentric contraction should also be ascertained. We have found that most athletes experience greater pain when landing from a jump or immediately prior to take-off following the eccentric preparatory phase (Fig. 5.3). Pain after stair-climbing (both up and down), as well as during prolonged sitting, has been described in cases of patellar tendinitis.

### Tenderness

Palpation of the likely painful site, as determined by the patient's age and description, often reveals tenderness. This sign confirms the diagnosis of patellar tendinitis. Most commonly, pain is felt at the inferior pole of the patella and is usually medial. Some postulated reasons for the predominance of medial pain (and therefore medial lesions in the tendon) are the oblique pole of the vastus medialis obliquus and the valgus alignment of the knee.

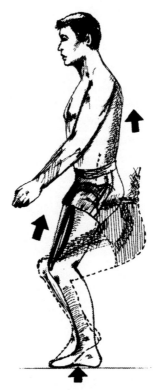

**Fig. 5.3 The largest forces occur during the eccentric phase of landing from a jump.**

## Inflammation

Pain is a result of inflammation. Sometimes it is possible to palpate increased temperature and some soft tissue swelling. These signs are uncommon, however, and usually appear in the long standing cases in which nearby soft tissues, such as the infrapatellar fat pad, are also irritated.

## Stiffness

Patients commonly complain of stiffness if they keep the knee in one position for any length of time and particularly if that position is knee flexion, such as that required by sitting in a car or in a movie.

Other signs

The patient with Osgood-Schlatter's disease may demonstrate an enlarged tibial tubercle. Usually this is found in the older adolescent who has had symptoms for a long time or who has stopped growing. Another sign is a decline in athletic performance, such as decreased vertical jumping ability. One very helpful sign is the occurrence of pain followed by a rapid eccentric force applied to the extended leg. This is easily reproduced by applying manual pressure to the limb, as shown in Fig. 5.4.

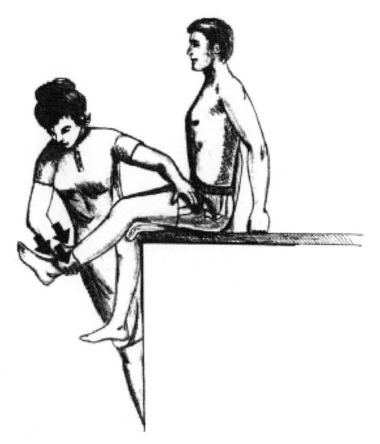

**Fig. 5.4 Have the patient extend the leg, then suddenly apply downward pressure. This may reproduce the symptoms.**

## Classification

Blazina *et al.* (1973) proposed the first classification of patellar tendon disorders (Table 5.1). We prefer to use the classification described in Chapters 3 and 4 and shown again in Table 5.2.

**Table 5.1  Classification of patellar disorder after (Blazina _et al._ 1973).**

| | |
|---|---|
| Stage 1 | Pain only after sports activity |
| Stage 2 | Pain at the beginning of sports activity disappearing after warm-up and reappearing with fatigue |
| Stage 3 | Constant pain at rest and during activity; patient unable to participate in sports at previous level |
| Stage 4 | Complete rupture of patellar tendon |

**Table 5.2  Classification of patellar disorder according to pain.**

| | |
|---|---|
| Level 1 | No pain |
| Level 2 | Pain with extreme exertion only; does not hinder sports performance and disappears when activity stops |
| Level 3 | Pain with exertion, remains 1 to 2 hours afterwards |
| Level 4 | Pain during any athletic activity, lasts 4 to 6 hours afterwards, increases throughout activity; performance level decreased |
| Level 5 | Pain starts immediately after activity commences, causes withdrawal from activity |
| Level 6 | Pain during daily activities; patient unable to participate in any sports |

## Etiology

A discussion of the etiology of patellar tendinitis requires consideration of the forces applied to the tendon during various activities (Table 5.3). There is considerable variation in some of these forces, but large stresses that nearly match the maximum tensile strength of the tendon can take place in normal athletic activities such as running.

**Table 5.3  Forces in patellar tendon during activities.**

| Activity | Force (N) | Stress (MPa) |
|---|---|---|
| Running | 7500–9000 | 37.5–45.0 |
| Kicking | 5200 | 26.0 |
| Jumping (landing) | 8000 | 40.0 |
| Jumping (take off) | 2500 | 12.5 |
| Walking | 500 | 2.5 |

A few studies provide valuable insight into the role of eccentric movement in patellar tendinitis. Wahrenberg _et al._ (1978) recorded the tendon tension force and electromyograph activity during the kicking of a soccer ball and found that the maximum tension occurred very early in the movement, when the initial knee flexion changed to extension, long before the ball was hit. This coincided with the peak of quadriceps EMG activity. This study points out that a force of 5200 N, the highest value obtained, corresponds to seven times body weight and this tensile force is generated in a freely moving limb. Repetition of such forces may result in tendinitis.

In activities involving weight bearing, such as running and jumping, there is a potential for even greater forces, especially with rapid motions. Adding extra weight naturally increases the force. Zernicke *et al.* (1977) were able to obtain data concerning the force that produced tendon rupture in a weightlifter. The athlete suffered a patellar tendon rupture during the filming of a 175 kg lift. They estimated the patellar tendon tension at the time of rupture to be 14 500 N, or more than 17 times the lifter's body weight. Furthermore, the rupture took place at the peak in the knee joint moment that occurred as the lifter stopped the downward motion of his body and the weight.

This article provides one of the few examples in which the magnitude of load and the loading rate have been estimated during an actual injury. Clearly, humans cannot approach maximum loading conditions experimentally (Fig. 5.5). Richards *et al.* (1996) found that in national class volleyball players, the average ground reaction force during landing from a spike jump was 9.5 times the player's body weight. One player had a recording for one trial that was 11.6 times body weight (10 397 N).

The magnitudes of these forces seem to indicate that the patellar tendon is frequently subjected to loads approaching maximum during athletic activities. In addition, these loads are repeated. This cyclic loading reduces the ability of the tendon to elongate because it is unable to restore its molecular

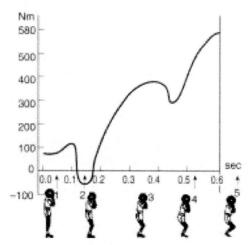

**Fig. 5.5** A knee-joint moment–time curve during a lift in which the patellar tendon ruptured. Forces were estimated at greater that 17 times body weight when the rupture occurred. Redrawn with permission from Zernicke, R. F., Garhammer, J., and Jobe, F. W. Human patella-tendon rupture. *J. Bone Joint Surg.* (*Am*), 59, (2), 179–83, 1977.

structure (Krahl 1976). Thus the tendon, which is perfectly elastic only in the area of 3–4% elongation caused by loads of less than one quarter of the maximum, may suffer microtears. It was previously thought (Elliott 1965) that tendons were probably not stressed to more than one quarter of their maximum tensile strength *in vivo*; however, more recent evidence suggests that near maximal forces are applied regularly.

We believe that eccentric movement is the major etiologic factor in patellar tendinitis, because of the higher patellar tendon tensions associated with eccentric contraction. This theory originates from patients statements describing maximum discomfort while landing from a jump or during rapid backward movement, as in tennis, and is supported by experimental evidence such as that of Wahrenberg *et al.* (1978), and Zernicke *et al.* (1977). Other proposed etiologic factors include the type of training (e.g. jumping), time spent training (number of sessions per week), and playing surface (harder surfaces increase the risk of tendinitis).

Recent studies have attempted to look at risk factors for patellar tendon dysfunction in volleyball players. Richards *et al.* (1996) were able to predict with 80% accuracy which players had pain at the time of testing, based on their analysis of such variables as ground reaction force and flexion angle of the knee during landing. One can extrapolate from their work that there is an optimal biomechanical technique for jumping with regards to avoiding patellar tendon symptoms. If this can be determined and taught, it would be an excellent way of preventing injury in this population. Lian *et al.* (1996) found that volleyball players with patellar tendon pain performed better in jumping tests (especially eccentric jumping) than asymptomatic controls. This is more likely to be cause than effect, and the authors concluded that players who jump well load their tendons more than others.

## Differential diagnosis

Knee joint complaints are probably most common in athletes and can easily be confusing to the inexperienced examiner. A careful history usually enables a tentative diagnosis to be made which can be confirmed by physical examination. The following are some conditions that may be mistaken for patellar tendinitis.

### Patello-femoral arthrosis

Patello-femoral arthrosis is easily confused with patellar tendinitis because of its similarity and symptoms—pain on squatting and jumping, stiffness after sitting, and so on. However, unlike tendinitis, there is no point tenderness at the usual sites of patellar tendinitis, nor is pain specific to eccentric activities. Quadriceps wasting is usually much more obvious in cases involving the patello-femoral joint.

## Meniscal tear

The history of this injury is different from that of tendinitis. A rotational injury is involved in most meniscal lesions. Locking and joint effusion are characteristic, and tenderness is present along the joint line. Giving way may be seen in the presence of jumper's knee, but should not be confused with true mechanical locking in which the patient is unable to extend the knee. Joint line tenderness will not be seen in jumper's knee.

## Infrapatellar fat pad inflammation (Hoffa's disease)

The infrapatellar fat pad can be irritated through overuse or following direct pressure on the anterior infrapatellar aspect of the knee. The symptoms mimic those of patello-femoral arthrosis and patellar tendinitis, but usually can be distinguished by the presence of pain when the fat pad is gently squeezed between the fingers and thumb. Swelling of the fat pad may also be evident.

## Bursitis

Of the numerous bursae around the knee, four are related to the quadriceps muscle (Fig. 5.6):

- suprapatellar bursa: between the anterior surface of the lower femur and the deep surface of the quadriceps;
- subcutaneous prepatellar bursa: between the lower part of the patella and the skin;
- subcutaneous infrapatellar bursa: between the lower part of the tibial tuberosity and the skin;
- deep infrapatellar bursa: between the patellar tendon and the tibia.

Bursitis can be easily confused with patellar tendinitis, especially in the case of deep infrapatellar bursitis, since tension in the tendon will compress the bursa and cause pain. Tenderness with pressure on the tibial tubercle is present. Since this site is uncommon for tendinitis beyond the adolescent years, one can suspect bursitis in older patients.

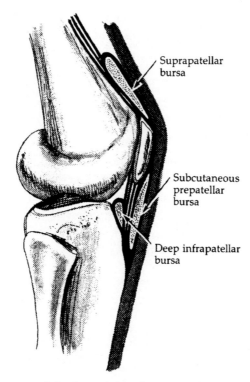

**Fig. 5.6  Bursae around the knee joint that may mimic patellar tendinitis.**

## Imaging

Since the first edition of this book, there have been numerous publications regarding the use of imaging studies in the diagnosis of patellar tendinitis. Ultrasound and magnetic resonance imaging (MRI) have been shown to be of particular value.

### X-rays

Soft tissue swelling is difficult to assess on some plain X-rays, and as such, they are not very useful in acute cases. In chronic cases, calcification of the tendon, elongation of the lower pole of the patella, and periosteal reaction of the lower patellar pole may all be seen. X-rays may help with the differential diagnosis (for example patello-femoral arthrosis), but are probably not mandatory if the history and physical are clearly diagnostic. X-rays should be obtained before surgery to look for calcific nodules that should be included in the excision of the area of tendinosis.

## Ultrasound

As the patellar tendon is a subcutaneous soft tissue structure, ultrasound should be quite good at detecting structural changes in the tendon; and indeed this is so. Numerous changes are seen in patellar tendinitis, including: (1) homogeneous thickening (thought to be due to peritendinous swelling); (2) hypoechoic areas (tendinosis, especially mucinous degeneration or cysts), (3) hyperechoic areas (calcific tendinosis).

Fritschy and deGautard (1988) attempt to predict treatment outcomes based on ultrasound appearance of the tendon, suggesting that more involved tendons with a thickened heterogenous appearance will require surgery for successful treatment. Khan *et al*. (1996) found an 18% incidence of degenerative changes in the ultrasounds of a control group, thus underscoring the fact that these changes are prevalent and may be subclinical and asymptomatic. Needless to say, we should be treating symptoms and not ultrasound findings. There are no studies that support ultrasound as a screening tool in at risk populations.

## Computed tomography (CT)

CT has largely been supplanted by MRI, as MRI is superior in imaging soft tissues. Ultrasound is probably more accurate as well.

## Magnetic resonance imaging (MRI)

MRI has shown good correlation with clinical and histological findings. The classic picture of tendinitis on MRI is that of increased signal intensity near the distal pole of the patella, with an increased anteroposterior diameter of the tendon proximally (less than 7 mm is considered normal). Indistinct posterior tendon margins and lesions in the medial and central one third of the proximal tendon are also characteristic (el-Khoury *et al*. 1992; McLoughlin *et al*. 1995).

Ultrasound and MRI have emerged as the imaging modalities of choice, with either one providing good diagnostic ability. The decision to select one over the other should be based on local factors such as cost, availability, and expertise available in interpretation. The role of these studies should be confirmatory or staging, with clinical findings being paramount to treatment decisions.

## Treatment

### General

The treatment of patellar tendinitis, for most clinicians, is no less frustrating than that of Achilles tendinitis, and the same variety of methods have been developed.

Frequently, cast immobilization is used to afford a period of rest for the tendon. This usually follows other conservative treatment measures such as stretching exercises, ultrasound, deep friction massage, knee supports, oral anti-inflammatory agents, and abstinence from sports. If a cast is applied, symptoms have usually disappeared by the time the cast is removed. Unfortunately they soon recur, since loads of the same magnitude are being applied to a tendon that has been weakened by immobility. Furthermore, quadriceps and calf muscle atrophy, and joint stiffness must be dealt with. The basic outline for the conservative treatment of patellar tendinitis is presented in Table 5.4, which follows Blazina *et al.*'s (1973) classification system.

**Table 5.4  Conservative treatment program for patellar tendinitis.**

| Stage 1 | Adequate warming up (5 to 10 minutes of push-ups, sit-ups, etc.) |
|---|---|
| | Ice after activity |
| | Local anti-inflammatory treatment and anti-inflammatory drugs for several weeks |
| | Physiotherapy, including isometric quadriceps exercises |
| | Elastic knee support |
| Stage 2 | Same as stage 1 |
| | Some form of heat before activity |
| | Period of rest |
| Stage 3 | Same as stage 2 but also prolonged period of rest |
| | If conservative treatment fails, abstinence from sports or surgery |
| Stage 4 | Primary repair of tendon |

The use of cast immobilization is decreasing as more people realize that it extends an already long period of immobility and gives only temporary relief of symptoms (Martens *et al.* 1982).

The use of steroid injections is also discouraged because of the danger of tendon rupture. Steroid injections provide temporary pain relief but cause mechanical damage to the tendon (see Chapter 2). In many studies of patients whose tendons rupture, a history of previous cortisone (steroid) injections has been noted. The absence of symptoms frequently causes the athlete to perform beyond his or her physical limits, thereby increasing the likelihood of further damage to the tendon.

Surgery is also becoming less popular as a treatment method, except in cases of tendon rupture, where it is essential. Typically, surgery is recommended for patients with pain preventing activity (Blazina *et al.*, Stage 3), of long standing duration (greater that 6–12 months), and non-responsive to conservative treatment. Surgery usually involves resection of the degenerated or necrotic tendon tissue, with or without drilling of the inferior pole of the patella to stimulate the growth of new blood vessels. This treatment is usually followed by a period of immobilization (4 to 6 weeks) and 3 to 8 months of rehabilitation. While some authors claim excellent results after surgical treatment (Blazina *et al.* 1973; Martens *et al.* 1982; Karlsson *et al.* 1991; Popp *et al.* 1997) no controlled studies comparing a treatment identical with the one that follows surgery have been performed. It seems quite plausible that over a four month period of rest from sports, considerable improvement in symptoms will occur.

## The eccentric exercise program

Despite the success or failure of other treatment methods, the fact remains that the tendon is damaged when its tensile strength is exceeded, thus a treatment program to increase this tensile strength should make the tendon less susceptible to injury. We agree with many of the conservative treatment methods, particularly the importance of warm-up and flexibility exercises before activity and ice application after. Flexibility training is important because not only does it increase the elasticity of the muscle-tendon unit, but it may also increase the tensile strength of the tendon. However, the main advantage of the eccentric exercise program is that neither immobilization nor rest is necessary, except in very painful cases where athletic activity is impossible. Most athletes with patellar tendinitis have very tight quadriceps (Fig. 5.7) which may be an etiologic factor.

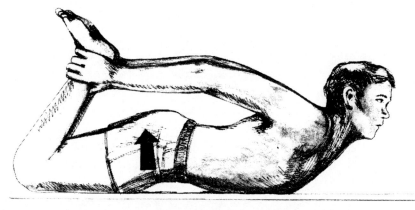

**Fig. 5.7 Testing for the quadriceps tightness: if hip begins to flex as foot is pulled toward buttocks, then these muscles are tight.**

The basis of the program is to use activities that place maximal stress on the tendon in order to increase its tensile strength. For the patellar tendon this is most readily achieved by having the patient drop to a semi squatting position (Fig. 5.8). The stress on the tendon is increased by adding weight resistance or dropping at a faster rate. It is not possible to assess the loads on the patellar tendon with these variations quantitatively, but the patient's discomfort acts as a monitor. The program is outlined in Table 5.5.

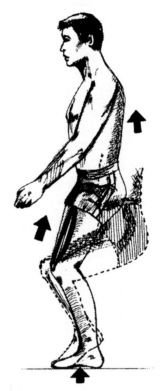

**Fig. 5.8  Patient drops (or lowers) to a semi-squatting position.**

'Slow movement' during the eccentric program means a controlled lowering of the body to the semi-crouched position and returning it to upright at the same speed. Speed is increased by allowing the body weight to drop more and more rapidly. Finally, patients should be able to allow their body weight to drop freely and stop the movement with eccentric quadriceps contraction. We call this motion drop and stop. The patient must understand that the sudden reversal of downward motion is the important feature of the program. As previously explained, no resistance is added until the patient can drop and stop with little or no discomfort. Then the program continues (Fig. 5.9).

The load on the tendon can be increased further if the athlete drops from a height and the load increases with the drop rate. We have not yet had to incorporate this into our program, but this revision may be more feasible than

**Table 5.5 Eccentric exercise program for jumper's knee.**

1. Warm-up
   a. General, whole-body warm-up
   b. Exercise not involving knee extension
   c. Sufficient when sweating is elicited
2. Stretching
   a. Static stretch of quadriceps and hamstrings
   b. Hold at least 30 seconds
   c. Repeat 3 times
3. Main program
   a. Squatting movements
   b. Focusing primarily on the rapid deceleration phase between the
      downward and upward movement phase
      Week 1: No added resistance on days 1 and 2 (slow); days 3 to 7
      (progressively faster)
      Week 2: Add resistance (10% body weight)
      Weeks 3 to 6: Add 4.5–13.5 kg progressively
   c. Do three sets of 10 repetitions once daily
   d. After 6 weeks, three sets of 10 three times weekly
4. Warm-down
   a. Static stretch as in item 2
5. Ice
   a. Ice on patellar tendon for 5 minutes after program
6. Optional support
   a. Apply tensor bandage support if desired

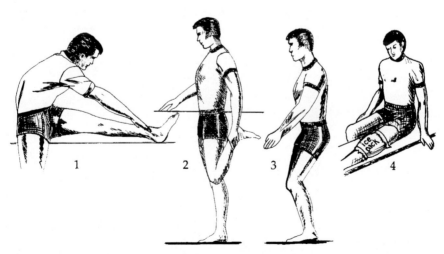

**Fig. 5.9 The stages of the exercise program: (1) stretch, (2) stretch quads, (3) eccentric exercise, (4) ice (after stretching again).**

the addition of heavy weights to the shoulders. Also, the movement more closely resembles that used in volleyball and basketball and can be combined with subsequent concentric contraction to practice vertical jumping. Indeed, this method is used by many gymnastic and volleyball coaches to improve jumping ability. This technique is called depth jumping or plyometrics (Kovalev 1981; Suwara 1979).

Jensen and Di Fabio (1989) prospectively evaluated eccentric exercise on quadriceps strength in patients with patellar tendinitis and normal controls. They found that both normals and tendinitis patients increased their quadriceps strength (significant increases in normals only) with eccentric exercises using a dynamometer versus groups of normals and tendinitis patients who performed home stretching exercises only. This study reinforces the fact that eccentric exercise strengthens muscle (and tendon by inference). However, the fact that the increase seen in tendinitis patients was not significant is concerning. It was attributed in the article to the pain level experienced by the tendinitis patients. This illustrates the importance of the program as a whole (warm-up exercises, stretching, ice treatment) and not just the exercises themselves. Pain relief is essential to treatment, and should be accomplished with the judicious use of rest, medications, and treatment modalities (as outlined in Chapter 2). Another essential feature of the program is that the progression exercise intensity should be based on the patient's symptoms and not the time elapsed since the treatment started (as in Jensen and Di Fabio 1989). This may explain why pain was still a prominent feature for these patients at eight weeks.

The rate of failure of conservative treatment for patellar tendinitis (and hence the need for surgery) has been estimated between 16% and 33% for chronic cases. Eccentric exercise was not a part of the conservative treatment program in these studies; and these rates may be drastically decreased with the eccentric exercise program, thus obviating the need for surgery in many cases.

# 6 Humeral epicondylitis

Tennis elbow refers to a variety of disorders involving the elbow joint. In fact, more than twenty-five lesions of this kind have been listed in the literature, including bursitis, arthritis, and neuritis (Priest 1976). The majority of authors, however, seem to agree with Nirschl (1974) who states, 'It is our conclusion that the pathological entity itself is a granulation response to microrupture of the extensor carpi radialis brevis and communis aponeurosis at the lateral epicondyle, as well as the subtendinous triangular space at the lateral epicondyle'. Nirschl has since coined the term 'angiofibroblastic hyperplasia' to describe these characteristic changes.

We concur with this opinion, but narrow our definition of tennis elbow to elbow pain that can be related to the extensor movements of the wrist joint. These extensors commonly attach to the lateral epicondyle, so the term lateral epicondylitis is preferable to tennis elbow, especially since the syndrome commonly occurs in non athletes whose occupations involved repeated gripping activities, such as carpenters, fishers, and homemakers.

Medial epicondylitis refers to elbow pain due to involvement of the wrist flexors and pronator teres, that attach to the medial epicondyle, and medial epicondylitis exhibits similar changes to those seen in lateral epicondylitis. However, it is, far less common, representing only 10–20% of all epicondylitis diagnoses (Plancher *et al.* 1996). For the sake of simplicity, we will use the term epicondylitis for both medial and lateral tendinopathies of the elbow unless otherwise specified.

## Structure and function

The lateral epicondyle of the humerus is a point of origin for the wrist extensors, including extensor carpi radialis longus, extensor carpi radialis brevis, extensor digitorum, and extensor digiti minimi. These muscles attach jointly to the lateral epicondyle via a tendinous expansion known as the common extensor tendon, or extensor aponeurosis (Fig. 6.1). In addition, the supinator muscle partially attaches to the lateral epicondyle and lies underneath the wrist extensor muscles mentioned above (Fig. 6.2).

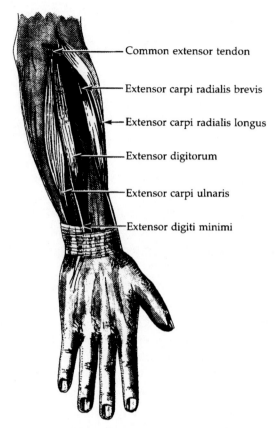

Common extensor tendon

Extensor carpi radialis brevis

Extensor carpi radialis longus

Extensor digitorum

Extensor carpi ulnaris

Extensor digiti minimi

**Fig. 6.1  The forearm muscles (extensor) that attach to the lateral epicondyle.**

These muscles act to extend the wrist and, in the case of the supinator, to supinate the forearm. The usual activity of the wrist extensors is a synergistic one, whereby the finger flexors contract simultaneously with wrist extension. The positioning of the wrist in extension allows a much more powerful grip. You can easily confirm this by attempting to grip an object, first with the wrist extended and then with it flexed. This stabilizing action of the wrist extensors means they are active in virtually all activities requiring use of the hand. The demand increases when stronger gripping is required, whether to hit a backhand playing tennis or to use a chain saw.

The medial epicondyle is the origin for the wrist flexors. These muscles include flexor carpi radialis, palmaris longus, flexor carpi ulnaris, and flexor digitorum superficialis, and they share a common origin with the pronator teres, the common flexor tendon.

These muscles act to flex the wrist, and the fingers in the case of the flexor digitorum superficialis, and pronate the forearm. Wrist flexors are synergistic with finger extensors so these muscles do not come into play during grip, which accounts for the decreased incidence of medial elbow tendinopathy.

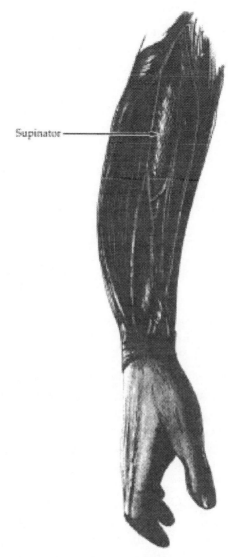

Supinator

**Fig. 6.2 Supinator lies beneath the wrist extensors, but is intimately connected.**

Valgus overload injuries (such as throwing) and impact activities (such as golf, tennis) are causative factors, as are repetitive tasks such as using a screwdriver or a hammer.

The ultrastructure of the normal common extensor and flexor tendons can be presumed to be similar to that of other tendinous structures, though it is shorter and thinner than the tendons in the other clinical situations described.

## Etiology and mechanics

Despite hundreds of articles throughout the last century, the precise etiology of epicondylitis remains to be clarified. This is the result of the wide range of sources to which the symptoms are attributed. However, there is agreement, that the etiology is probably multifactorial, including one or more of the following:

- massive overload of the flexor-pronator or extensor muscles
- multiple repetition of movement
- quality of tissue
- age
- potential hormonal imbalance (in females)
- strength
- endurance
- flexibility
- mechanics of joint design
- equipment
- skill level.

As in the other cases of chronic tendinitis, the basic etiology of the lesion is the application of forces that exceed the tensile strength of the common extensor or flexor tendons. These forces are produced by the wrist extensors or flexors, so any repeated movements involving marked flexion or extension movements of the wrist may be responsible. If the tendon is weakened because of previous injury, inflammation, hormonal imbalance, or nutritional deficiency, then it may be more susceptible to damage. Age-related changes may be classified as previous injury, since they are degenerative changes related to repeated microtraumas. This accounts for the high incidence of symptoms in individuals between the ages of thirty-five and fifty years.

It has been estimated that up to 50% of tennis players will develop epicondylitis in their playing lifetime (Kamien 1990), but depending on the referral population, only 5% of epicondylitis cases can be attributed to tennis (Ernst 1992). The study by Hutchinson et al. (1995) further underscores the roles that aging and degeneration play in the etiology of epicondylitis as they found a prevalence of only 1.2% in elite under-18 tennis players at a national tennis championship over a six year period.

Much research has been performed to investigate the pathogenesis of epicondylitis in tennis players. EMG studies (Morris et al. 1989) have demonstrated that the wrist extensors are active during the forehand and backhand strokes, as well as during serves. Thus the common extensor origin is at risk during all parts of the game. Numerous risk factors have been defined for the production of epicondylitis in tennis players:

- hitting the ball off centre (outside the 'sweet spot');
- pre-impact force on the racquet handle (strength of grip);
- incorrect grip size (too large or too small);
- excessive string tension;
- racquet design (higher resonance frequency decreases transmitted vibrations to the upper extremity);
- hitting wet balls, or hitting on a windy day;
- incorrect stroke technique.

The common denominator in all these risk factors is that they place undue stress on the muscles of the lateral (and occasionally medial) epicondyle to control joint moments or transmitted arm vibrations. This stress is in the form of eccentric overload, as (in the case of a backhand) the wrist flexes at the time of ball striking and the wrist extensors are called upon to control the flexion moment produced at the wrist. Knudson and Blackwell (1997) found that the wrist extensor moment was negative (that is a flexion moment) for amateur tennis players with lateral epicondylitis using a one-hand backhand, whereas it was positive for asymptomatic amateurs and professionals with a one-hand backhand (significant differences were only noted between the amateurs with lateral epicondylitis and the professionals). This study illustrates the role of eccentric overload in the pathogenesis of epicondylitis. In the beginner, off-centre hits and incorrect technique are common, and a tennis coach may be every bit as helpful as a doctor (if not more) in dealing with these risk factors.

The classic stroke flaw leading to extensor overload is a leading-elbow backhand (Fig. 6.3), where at the time of contact, the elbow is ahead of the tennis racquet. A two-hand backhand has been advocated as one way to reduce the incidence of lateral epicondylitis, as there is more support for the racket and it helps to eliminate stroke flaws, although no difference in wrist extensor EMG activity was seen in professional tennis players using one and two-hand backhands (Giangarra *et al.* 1993). The beneficial effect of the two-hand backhand may be more pronounced in less skilled players however, as professionals have the wrist extensor strength and technique to minimize stress on the common extensor tendon. The reader is referred to the work of Ilfeld (1992) for an elegant and more detailed discussion regarding the role of technique errors in the genesis of medial and lateral epicondylitis.

Another sport particularly likely to cause epicondylitis is squash. The racket grip is much smaller, and wrist extensor action is required more constantly since the wrist should be cocked throughout both forehand and backhand strokes. Players with a 'wristy backhand' or who are playing a lob from the front of the court are especially vulnerable. Nonetheless, fewer squash players are afflicted, probably because of the lighter rackets used. Badminton players fall in the same category as squash players. They use even more wrist

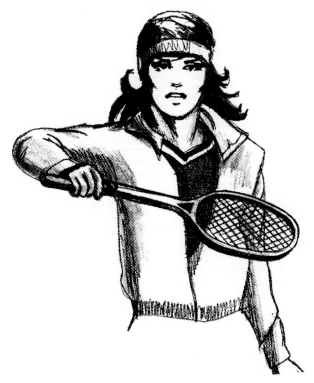

Fig. 6.3  The leading-elbow stroke.

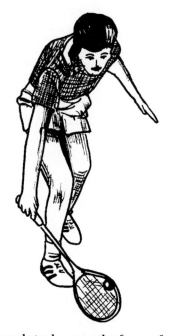

Fig. 6.4  A backhand stroke near the front of the squash court.

extension, but the racquet is very light so they are less susceptible to lateral epicondylitis (Fig. 6.4).

The principles described for tennis players apply to others as well: repeated loading over an extended period or a sudden increase in use of the wrist extensors (such as in renovating a house) may cause tennis elbow in non-athletes.

## Signs and symptoms

The symptoms of lateral epicondylitis are pain during strong gripping actions and weakness of the grip as a result of pain. The signs are tenderness with pressure on the point of the lateral epicondyle, pain and weakness with resisted wrist extension, and pain on stretching of the wrist extensors (Fig. 6.5). Medial epicondylitis has a similar presentation, with pain on activities that stress the flexors and pronators and weak grasp seen due to pain. Physical examination reveals point tenderness over the medial epicondyle, pain on resisted pronation and wrist flexion, and pain on stretching the wrist flexors.

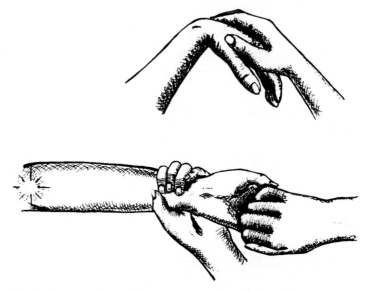

**Fig. 6.5 Pain is experienced on passive stretch and on resisted wrist extension.**

It is important to assess the status of the ulnar nerve and the valgus stability of the elbow in patients with medial epicondylitis, as the presence of ulnar neuritis or valgus instability will significantly affect treatment and outcomes of treatment. The estimate of the number of patients who have associated ulnar nerve pathology ranges from 24–60% in those with medial epicondylitis who progress to need surgery (Ollivierre *et al.* 1995; Kurvers and Verhaar 1995).

## Imaging

Plain X-rays are used mainly to exclude other diagnoses, such as tumor or fracture. Peri-epicondylar calcification may be seen in 5–20% of epicondylitis cases, but is of no prognostic value.

Ultrasound has been used, but has been largely supplanted by MRI for its better quality images and the ability to assess other structures. MRI has been shown to have good correlation with surgical findings (Potter *et al*. 1995) and has characteristic changes, including:

1. Normal or increased tendon thickness with increased signal intensity on T-1 images.
2. Tears outlined by bright signal (fluid) on T-2 images.
3. Peritendinitis (high signal surrounding tendon on T-2 images).
4. Calcification (focus of black signal) within an abnormal tendon.

However, in the vast majority of patients this is a diagnosis of history and physical exam. Imaging studies should be reserved for when there is doubt as to the diagnosis.

## Differential diagnosis

Intra-articular problems may have a similar presentation to tennis elbow, and can be evaluated by diagnostic intra-articular injection of local anaesthetic. Neurologic problems may be evaluated using EMG, which can be especially helpful in determining the status of the ulnar nerve. EMG is reported to be less helpful in evaluating the posterior inner osseous nerve. Major differential diagnoses to be aware of include:

Lateral
1. Posterior interosseous nerve syndrome.
2. Posterolateral rotary instability of the elbow joint.
Medial
1. Ulnar neuritis.
2. Valgus instability.

The existence of posterior interosseous nerve entrapment has been questioned by some authors, as it has been noted that releasing the supinator also relieves tension on the extensor carpi radialis brevis (site of most lateral epicondylitis), as they have a common origin. Thus, perhaps it is completing the release rather than decompressing the posterior interosseous nerve that gives relief in persistent cases treated as posterior interosseous nerve entrapment.

Organ *et al.* (1997) indirectly support this theory, as they found that at the time of salvage surgery for lateral epicondylitis, the symptoms of 97% (34 out of 35) of cases could have been attributed to residual tendinosis found at surgical exploration.


## Pathology

The use of surgery as a treatment for resistant cases of lateral epicondylitis offers a means by which the pathologic changes occurring in the common extensor tendon (and flexor pronator mass) may be examined. Such reports are numerous in the literature. Specimens of excised tissue show scattered areas of thinning and fibrilation of fibre bundles, with microruptures of tendinous bundles. These microruptures were not discernable during surgery, but are characterized by a break in the axial arrangement of the fibres, with the break filled by amorphus debris. They are accompanied by fibroblastic cell reaction and vascular proliferation. You will recognize this as the response to tendon injury outlined in Chapter 2: Tendon overuse results in microscopic rupture and subsequent tendinous non-repair with immature tissue.

The most common locations for these pathologic changes are in the extensor carpi radialis brevis (ECRB) for lateral epicondylitis, and in the flexor carpi radialis (FCR) to pronator teres (PT) interval for medial epicondylitis (Table 6.1).


## Treatment

In view of the diversity of opinion regarding the etiology of tennis elbow, it is not surprising to find an equally vast array of treatment techniques. The list includes rest, cast immobilization, steroid injection, systemic anti-inflammatories, ice, ultrasound, heat, deep friction, manipulation, acupuncture, bracing and surgery. Laser therapy, pulsed electromagnetic fields, glycosaminoglycan injections, extra corporeal shock waves (lithotripsy), and even radiation therapy and botulinum toxin have been tried in conservative treatment regimes, but should **all** be considered experimental at this point. Although some of these methods may prove successful under certain circumstances, the very existence of such variety and the number of patients who have experienced many of, or all of, these treatment techniques should serve as convincing evidence that none is entirely successful.

At present, there are many articles of varying quality dealing with conservative treatment regimes and modalities. However, notable by its absence is

**Table 6.1  Structures described by various authors as being the underlying pathology in tennis elbow compiled by Cyriax (1936). It is just as diverse today.**

1. Traumatic periostitis
2. Arthritis, synovitis, sprain, adhesions, or torn capsule of the radiohumeral joint
3. Arthritis, synovitis, sprain, or adhesions of the radioulnar joint
4. Displaced, frayed, torn, or inflamed orbicular ligament
5. Sprained, torn radial collateral ligament
6. Inflamed radiohumeral bursa
7. Inflamed subcutaneous epicondylar bursa
8. Nipped synovial fringe in radiohumeral or radioulnar joint
9. Tear or fibrositis of extensor origin
10. Tear or fibrositis of supinator
11. Torn pronator teres
12. Torn extensor carpi radialis longus
13. Torn extensor carpi radialis brevis
14. Tear of brachioradialis
15. Tear of extensor digitorum communis
16. Myositis or tear of extensor muscles
17. Torn anconeus
18. Radial incongruence
19. Rheumatism, gout, influenzal sequelae, focal sepsis
20. Neuritis of radial, posterior interosseous, or antebrachial cutaneous nerves
21. Osteochondritis.

any study investigating the effect of an eccentric exercise program. Many of the treatments listed above can never be consistently successful because they address the symptoms of epicondylitis (pain) rather than the cause (eccentric overload of muscles). Without addressing the cause of the problem, other modes of treatment are doomed to failure, or to provide temporary relief at best, if the patient does not alter their activity level. Patients may not be willing or financially able to curtail their activities, and as such, return to full function should be the goal in every patient.

In his attempt to consolidate the various treatments, Nirschl (1974) presented a good review of treatment concepts:

1. Relief of acute inflammation.
2. Relief of chronic inflammation.
3. Increasing forearm muscle power, flexibility, and endurance.
4. Decreasing the moment of force at the elbow:  (a)  alter sport
                                                 (b)  change equipment
                                                 (c)  use an elbow support.
5.  Surgery, if conservative treatment fails.

Our treatment does not differ greatly from this regime. We advocate the liberal use of ice and sometimes oral anti-inflammatory drugs and corticosteroid injections to control inflammation. Brief periods of rest may be necessary in acute cases. The use of a forearm brace (Fig. 6.6) is also suggested to relieve

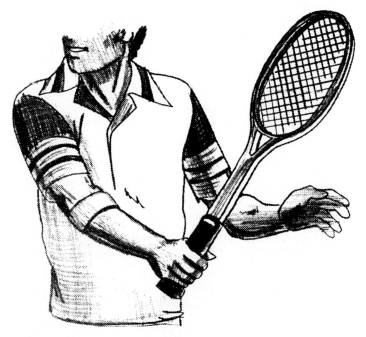

**Fig. 6.6  Use of a forearm band to relieve symptoms.**

symptoms during the treatment period. The exact mechanism of action of this brace is unclear, but it appears to function by providing a reactive counter-force against the contracting muscles and either spreads the force over a wider area, or decreases the contractile pull on the lateral epicondyle. The brace is applied snugly to the relaxed forearm, just prior to activity, and is removed immediately afterwards. Evidence in the literature regarding braces is also contradictory, with some studies showing no effect of braces on pain and grip strength (Wuori *et al.* 1998) or EMG activation of muscles (Glazebrook *et al.* 1994), whereas Burton (1985) found increased pain-free grip strength with two different types of bands. In addition, an air bladder type of forearm band was found to be more effective than standard bands in reducing EMG activity in healthy people (Snyder-Mackler and Epler 1989). The lack of clear consensus makes it impossible for us to offer any recommendations. The reader is left to his or her own judgement and experience to determine the place of forearm bands in the treatment armamentarium.

The main difference in our approach to the treatment of epicondylitis lies in our emphasis on exercise. This stems from the knowledge that decreased flexibility causes the muscles to be overstretched during eccentric contraction and overloading of the muscles is the most widely recognized factor in the etiology of the syndrome. Maximum strengthening of the muscle must necessarily include eccentric exercise, since this is the nature of the force producing the injury and since eccentric exercise produces greater tensile force on the tendon.

Control of loading on the muscle is carried out by altering the speed of movement or the amount of resistance. We suggest a starting weight of one kilogram (two pounds) (0.5 kg/1 lb for women) in acute cases, and 2.5 kg (five pounds) in less severe cases. Warm-up may be effectively provided by local heat application for a few minutes or via general body exercise.

The program we will describe below is specific for lateral epicondylitis but the principles may be applied to cases of medial epicondylitis as well. The patient stretches the wrist extensors by pronating the forearm with the elbow extended and then passively flexing the wrist. This flexing may be done with the opposite hand or by placing the flexed hand on the support of a suitable level (Fig. 6.7).

Following three 30 second stretches, the patient sits with the forearm supported so that the hand and weight are beyond the support. Then the weight may be lowered and raised freely. Again, the emphasis is on the change from downward to upward motion. The exercise is repeated thirty times, in three sets of ten (Fig. 6.8). The stretching exercises are repeated, and ice is applied to the lateral epicondyle. One very convenient method of doing this is to freeze a paper cup full of water and use this to rub gently over the area for five minutes. It may be placed back in the freezer and reused. Alternatively, an ice cube with a stick frozen inside it or crushed ice in a damp towel may be used (Fig. 6.9).

The entire session should take about twenty minutes and is to be carried out daily. As with Achilles and patellar tendinitides, it may be two or three weeks before symptoms begin to abate. During this interval, the patient should be checked regularly to ensure the program is done regularly and correctly, and progresses when indicated. The yardstick of discomfort (or absence of same) near the end of thirty repetitions, determines when the speed or resistance should be changed. This program can be quite easily adapted to medial epicondylitis by stretching and exercising the appropriate muscles of the medial epicondyle.

## Surgery

Surgery is often used as a last resort, after six to twelve months of conservative treatment has failed. It has been estimated that 5–10% of patients presented to a doctor will require surgical treatment of some sort, with the two major types of procedures being releases (open or percutaneous) and repairs

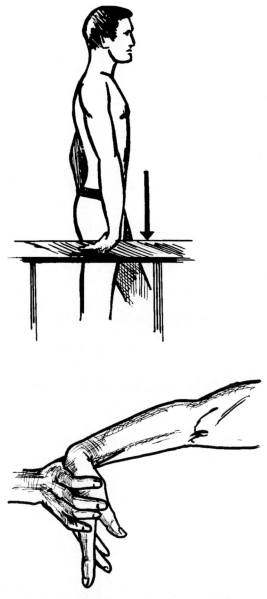

**Fig. 6.7 Stretching the wrist extensors.**

with resection of tendinosis. Denervation, distal lengthening, and intra-articular procedures have been described, but are not as popular or successful.

Releases involve simple transection of the affected tendon, with the premise that the tendon will heal in a lengthened position, thus lessening the stress across it. Avascular response will also be provoked by the insult, leading to better blood flow to the area and promoting healing. Good or excellent results, commonly defined as full function, with little or no pain and normal or near-normal grip strength, have been reported in more than 85–90% of

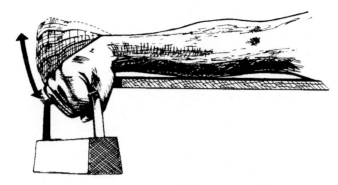

Fig. 6.8  With forearm supported, lower weight over the side.

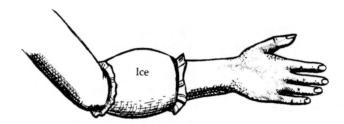

Fig. 6.9  Final stage: apply ice.

cases (Yerger and Turner 1985; Goldberg *et al.* 1988; Verhaar *et al.* 1993). Crit-
ics counter that simple release does not address the pathology, and may be
likely to cause damage, especially to the ulnar nerve and ulnar collateral ligament on the medial side. Organ *et al.*'s (1997) study showing that residual
disease is the main culprit in surgical failures is further argument against
simple release. In addition, some of the studies of simple release have shown
a prolonged time to healing which has been postulated to be due to the
natural history of the disease rather than any surgical intervention.

Resection and repair procedures advocated by Coonrad and Hooper (1973),
Nirschl and Pettrone (1979), and Vangsness and Jobe (1991) involved careful
dissection and excision of degenerative areas of tendinosis, followed by repair
of the common extensor (or flexor) origin. Success rates (good or excellent
results) of greater than 75% to 95% have been demonstrated. Others argue
that the more extensive release and morbidity with these procedures is not
necessary in the face of equal results with a less invasive procedure. Again, in
the absence of any comparative studies between the two procedures, no
definitive recommendations can be made.

The issue of the ulnar nerve and medial epicondylitis surgery deserves
mention. Both Kurvers and Verhaar (1995) and Gabel and Morrey (1995)
have found that ulnar nerve dysfunction negatively impacts prognosis after
surgery, and should be addressed at the time of surgery by either decompression and/or transposition. The clinician is therefore advised to look diligently

for ulnar nerve dysfunction prior to surgery for medial epicondylitis and address it, if present.

In review of the article by Ollivierre *et al.* (1995), it was stated that the post-operative rehabilitation is as important as the surgery. We concur with this statement, as we feel that even surgery cannot address the cause of epicondylitis (eccentric overload). The only way to strengthen the tendon so it can meet the demands placed upon it is exercise, which is most effectively performed with the eccentric exercise program.

# 7    Other tendinitides

There are numerous other tendinitides that can be equally difficult to treat. The purpose of this chapter is to review some of these disorders, their etiologies, and possible avenues of treatment. We do not advocate the use of eccentric exercises in treating all types of tendinitis and not all the clinical entities mentioned in this chapter are necessarily amenable to treatment with eccentric exercise. We present what we feel is the best method of treatment or the most widely used.

## Upper limb

### Shoulder and shoulder girdle

*Supraspinatus tendinitis*

This is the most common type of tendinitis in the upper limb. It occurs most frequently in swimmers and tennis players, or athletes in any sport requiring repeated overhead movement of the arm. Knowledge of the anatomy of the shoulder joint and supraspinatus tendon is essential for understanding this injury. The supraspinatus tendon passes beneath the acromion and inserts on the greater tuberosity of the humerus, passing beneath the coracoacromial ligament which forms a fibrous arch over the tendon. Between the tendon and the overlying structures is the subacromial bursa.

Repeated abduction of the shoulder, unless it is maintained in external rotation, causes impingement of the tendon within the very narrow space between the humerus and the overlying acromion and ligament. This disorder is often referred to as **impingement syndrome**. You can readily see how the freestyle stroke in swimming can cause this disorder, which has a second nickname, **swimmer's shoulder**.

It has long been orthopaedic dogma that supraspinatus tendinitis is an example of exogenous tendinitis (due to pressure and attrition from external sources). However, increasing evidence is accumulating that this is an endogenous tendinitis (an intrinsic tendon problem), or a tendinosis, as seen

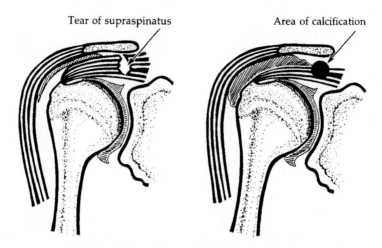

Tear of supraspinatus                                    Area of calcification

**Fig. 7.1  Sites of supraspinatus tendinitis.**

in the Achilles and patellar tendons (Fig. 7.1). Aging probably plays the most important part in rotator cuff degeneration, but tensile or compressive forces and subacromial inflammation may all be involved. The increased incidence of rotator cuff tears seen in anterior shoulder dislocations in patients over the age of forty, can be seen as indirect evidence that acute trauma can produce rotator cuff disruption, but most likely only in the setting of pre-existing degeneration, as seen in the Achilles and patellar tendons. It seems that the characteristic acromial spurring, seen with impingement syndrome, is being increasingly interpreted as a secondary effect of, rather than the cause of, impingement syndrome (Ozaki *et al.* 1988; Fukuda *et al.* 1990; Yazici *et al.* 1995).

If rotator cuff pathology is due to tendinosis, a logical next step is to develop an eccentric exercise program to strengthen the tendon to help control symptoms. It has been the senior author's (Stanish, W.D.) experience that shoulder arthroscopy has indirectly supported the concept of rotator cuff pathology as endogenous (rather than exogenous) tendinosis. We have observed patients with small, partial thickness articular surface tears of the rotator cuff on glenohumeral arthroscopy, who have an intact bursa surface of the cuff and pristine periosteum over the acromion on introduction of the arthroscope into the subacromial space. In this subgroup of patients, we have been debriding the articular surface tear and any reactive bursa, but leaving the acromion and coracoacromial ligament intact (rather than perform acromioplasty), as we feel that the acromion is not the problem. Altchek (1998) has proposed similar treatment in this subgroup he calls **athletic impingement**. However, he releases the coracoacromial ligament in this subgroup.

It is too soon to tell if this treatment method will prove to be better than the gold standard of acromioplasty, but this could be an interesting area of future research. It may be that the benefits of acromioplasty in the patient with an intact periosteum, are due more to the structured rehabilitation program that follows it, rather than the bone resection; if this is so, then an eccentric exercise program would probably be best for strengthening the tendon and eliminating the symptoms caused by tendinosis. The reader is referred to the work of Matsen *et al.* (1998) for an excellent comprehensive review of the concept of rotator cuff tendinosis and the pathogenesis of impingement syndrome.

*Bicipital tendinitis*

The long head of the biceps arises by long, narrow tendon from the superglenoid tubercle of the scapula. The long head passes through the shoulder joint and emerges from it to lie in the intertubercular sulcus (bicipital groove) where it is restrained by the transverse humeral ligament (Fig. 7.2), as well as

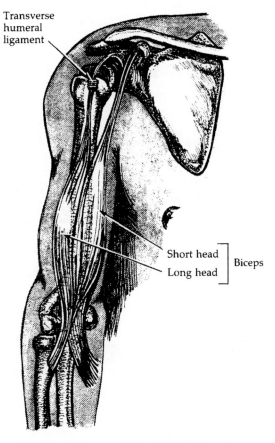

**Fig. 7.2 Anatomy of the bicipital tendon.**

the tendons of the rotator cuff, the coracohumeral ligament, and the superior glenohumeral ligament. Thus, it is subject to the same type of impingement as the supraspinatus tendon; indeed, it is common for biceps tendinitis to be associated with rotator cuff pathology. One distinguishing feature relates to internal and external rotation of the shoulder. During abduction, rotation is usually painful in cases of bicipital tendinitis, especially if the examiner applies slight pressure with the fingers to the tendon in its groove, while the arm is maneuvered passively. In patients with supraspinatus tendinitis, the internally rotated position may be painful, but this pain will disappear when the humerus is rotated outward because the greater tuberosity of the humerus no longer impinges on the acromion process.

The slight differences in the mechanics of these two types of tendinitis mean that bicipital tendinitis occurs more often in athletes who participate in sports involving throwing or paddling. Of course, bicipital tendinitis may occur in swimmers and other athletes as well, usually secondary to supraspinatus tendinitis since the ensuing inflammation may involve the nearby biceps.

Treatment is usually aimed at relieving the inflammation and pressure on the tendon by means of ice, anti-inflammatory drugs, or a steroid injection into the tendon sheath. These conservative methods are nearly always successful, providing the rotator cuff pathology has been dealt with as well.

## *Triceps tendinitis*

The attachment of the long head of the triceps to the infraglenoid tubercle of the scapula, where it blends into the capsule of the shoulder joint, is sometimes a site of triceps tendinitis. Pain is produced by vigorous throwing and can be reproduced during examination by forward flexing the shoulder with the elbow flexed and having the patient attempt to extend the elbow against resistance (Fig. 7.3).

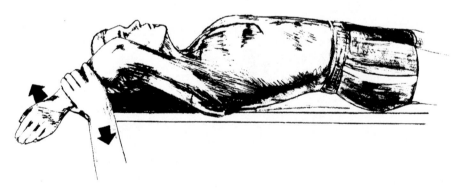

**Fig. 7.3 Stretching the triceps muscles (elbow must be flexed and shoulder extended as far as possible).**

The depth of this lesion and the covering of other muscles make it difficult to treat with ice, physiotherapy, or injection. Indeed, it proves very resistant to treatment and often recurs. We recommend strengthening the muscle eccentrically by having the patient exercise as shown in Fig. 7.4. The difficulty in performing these exercises adequately alone may make supervision and assistance from a therapist necessary.

### Other shoulder girdle muscles

The infraspinatus and teres minor may be injured during racket sports that require rotation of the shoulder, for example, squash. Treatment with stretching and resisted exercises, plus physiotherapeutic modalities to relieve symptoms, works rapidly in these cases. Less commonly, the scapular attachment of the teres major becomes painful, usually as a result of throwing. The symptoms are similar to those in triceps tendinitis, except that pain is reproduced by having the patient lie supine, with the arm abducted and fully externally rotated, and internally rotate the arm against manual resistance. In general, any muscle-tendon unit may give rise to pain, depending on the sport and the individual characteristics of the athlete. If doubt exists as to the muscle involved, careful positioning so that each muscle is placed in a lengthened position and made to contract against resistance can be helpful in identifying the specific muscle. These positions can be found in manuals of muscle testing (such as Daniels and Worthingham 1972).

### Elbow

The most common disorder here is, of course, humeral epicondylitis as discussed in Chapter 6.

### Wrist

Excessive, repetitive movements of, or pressure on, the wrist extensor tendons may inflame the tendon sheaths as they pass under the extensor retinaculum (Fig. 7.5). Most commonly affected are the tendons of the abductor pollicis longus and extensor pollicis brevis, which occupy the same synovial sheath and pass in a bony groove behind the radiostyloid process to form a sharp angle and insert on the thumb. Synovitis results from friction between the tendon and its sheath and the bony process and the overlying retinaculum. This is an example of exogenous tendinitis. The symptoms are aching discomfort over the styloid process, aggravated by movements of the wrist and thumb, and pain on stretching the tendons or resisted thumb abduction. Treatment usually consists of localized application of anti-inflammatory drugs, splinting of the wrist and thumb, and physiotherapy (usually ultrasound

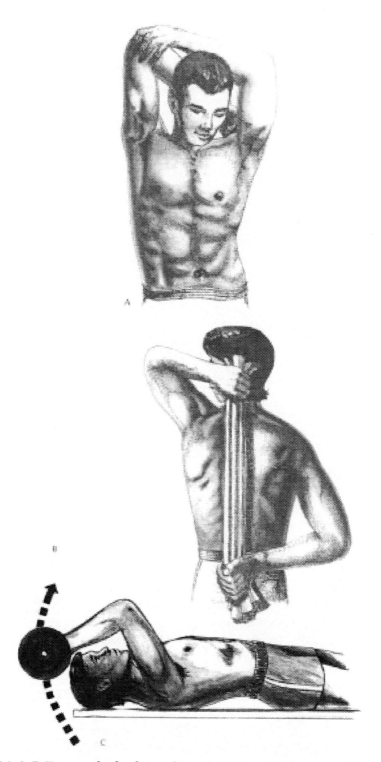

Fig. 7.4  A. B. Two methods of stretching the triceps. C. The eccentric exercise program.

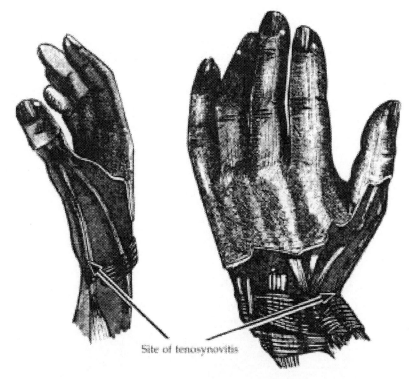

Site of tenosynovitis

**Fig. 7.5  De Quervain's syndrome due to increased pressure.**

and water). These measures are nearly always successful, although sometimes steroid injections or (more rarely) surgery may be necessary in very resistant cases.

## Lower Limb

The muscle-tendon units of the lower limb are subjected to greater force than those of the upper limb because of the larger masses (limb or body) that they must move. Also more regular activity is required of these muscles, both in daily activity (for example walking) and in sports. The most common tendinitides of the lower limb, Achilles tendinitis and jumper's knee, have already been discussed. The following are some of the other lower limb lesions that can occur, focusing on those in which eccentric contraction contributes to the etiology.

### Groin injury

Groin injuries include lesions in a number of muscles of the upper thigh, namely iliopsoas, rectus femoris, sartorius, pectineus, adductor longus,

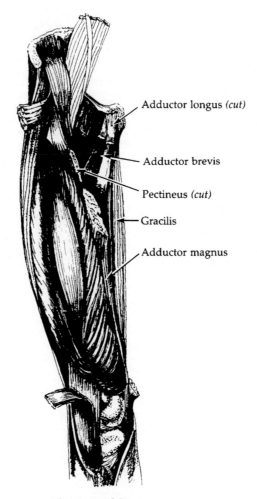

Adductor longus *(cut)*

Adductor brevis

Pectineus *(cut)*

Gracilis

Adductor magnus

**Fig. 7.6  Adductor muscles.**

adductor brevis, gracilis, and so on (Fig. 7.6). The action of these muscles (hip flexion and adduction) means that they are commonly used in kicking. They are also stretched when the hip joint is abducted and/or extended. Injury to these muscles occurs most frequently in soccer players, not an unusual finding in light of the action of these muscles and the use of the lower limbs in this sport. In kicking, first the hip is extended. Then this motion is arrested, and the hip is suddenly flexed (Fig. 7.7). At this point the iliopsoas and rectus femoris are contracting eccentrically. Also, the adductor muscles of the opposite limb must contract to maintain the horizontal position of the pelvis, especially if the player stops suddenly while running or changes direction. The fixing of the foot to the ground that occurs with the wearing of cleats (studs) may contribute to stretching of the adductor muscles. The second sport in which groin injuries commonly occur is ice hockey. The sliding of a skate laterally on the ice easily causes the adductor muscles to be over stretched.

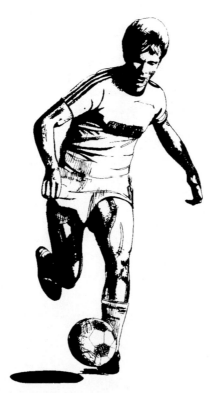

**Fig. 7.7  Leg changes from backward to forward, causing stretch in hip flexors and adductors.**

The symptoms of a **groin pull**, as these injuries are usually called, are pain on movements requiring stretch and/or contraction of the muscle (such as kicking or changing direction during skating or running). The pain may be severe enough to prevent the player from participating in sports. You can test clinically for this disorder by placing the hip in an abducted and slightly extended position and having the patient attempt both to flex and adduct the thigh simultaneously. It is important to have the patient initiate both muscle actions, since these movements performed singularly often will not cause symptoms (Fig. 7.8).

Many authors have implicated the adductor longus tendon as the most likely musculotendinous unit to become injured in the groin (Renstrom 1992; Karlsson *et al*. 1994; Gibbs 1994). In order to have a definitive diagnosis of the groin injury, it is important to remember to isolate muscles one at a time. Position them so they are stretched; then resist their contraction in length and position. Usually the affected muscle-tendon unit can be identified easily. Table 7.1 provides some common positions for testing various muscles of the thigh. Most physiotherapists are adept at selective muscle testing and should be consulted if any uncertainty remains.

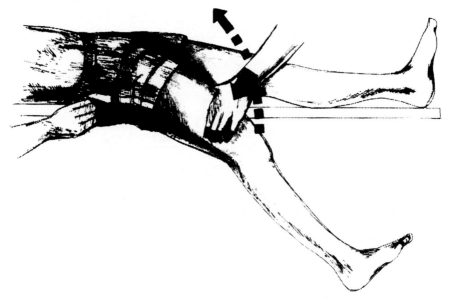

**Fig. 7.8 Resisting hip flexion/adduction. Examiner should stand beside patient for the best angle and to prevent falling.**

There are a number of differential diagnoses that should be considered when faced with a patient with groin injury. These include:

- Other musculotendinous units (rectus abdominus, rectus femoris, iliopsoas), which may be treated using the same principles;
- Hip joint pain (arthritis, AVN of the femoral head, stress fractures of the femoral neck);
- Pelvic pain (Sacro-iliac joint inflammation, stress fractures of the pubic rami, osteitis pubis);
- Hernias;
- Prostatitis;
- Nerve entrapment;
- Upper lumbar spine pathology;
- Tumors.

The history and physical exam should enable one to arrive at the correct diagnosis in most cases. The onset can be sudden or gradual, with a feeling of progressive tightness, and is exacerbated by activity and relieved with rest. The pain is characteristically located in the upper medial thigh, but may radiate distally. Tenderness over the proximal insertion and/or musculotendinous junction, and pain with resisted adduction are the hallmarks of the physical exam. Passive stretch of the adductors (hip abduction) may also reproduce the patient's symptoms.

For those cases that remain a diagnostic dilemma, imaging studies may be helpful in arriving at a diagnosis. Bone scans can help to localize areas of stress

**Table 7.1  Common positions for testing thigh muscles.**

| Muscle | Action | Position of patient | Test |
|---|---|---|---|
| Rectus femoris | Flex hip and extend knee | Supine | Flex hip with knee straight |
| Iliopsoas | Flex hip | Supine at edge of bed so hip can extend in neutral plane | Flex hip, allowing knee flexion |
| Sartorius | Flex hip and knee, externally rotate hip | Sitting over edge of plinth | Have patient flex hip while bringing knee to shoulder on same side |
| Pectineus, adductor brevis[a] | Adduct hip | Supine with leg slightly extended | Resist adduction in horizontal plane |
| Adductor longus, magnus | Adduct hip | Supine with leg abducted and knee flexed | Resist adduction in horizontal plane |
| Gracilis | Adduct hip, flex knee, medially rotate thigh | Supine with leg abducted and knee straight | Attempt to laterally rotate thigh while person resists (applying resistance at heel will bring knee flexion) |

[a] Since pectineus and adductor brevis are shorter muscles, less hip abduction is necessary to stretch them. Also, pectineus and adductor brevis originate more anteriorly on the pubis and so may be stretched farther by placing the hip in extension.

fracture or arthritis or avascular necrosis. Plain X-rays are useful only to exclude avulsion fractures and hip pathology; occasionally, calcification may be seen in the adductors. Kalebo *et al.* (1992) has found ultrasound to be useful and that it has good correlation with surgical findings. CT and MRI have also been advocated for imaging musculotendinous injuries in the groin (Speer *et al.* 1993). Ultrasound or MRI are acceptable choices for soft tissue imaging and the choice of one modality over the other should be based on local expertise and availability.

The combined flexion and adduction movement, with resistance added, is used in conservative treatment. Since it is difficult to apply external weight resistance (although ankle weights may be used), commonly the assistance of another person is required. Usually this is the therapist, since supervision is required and the exercise will be quite painful if it is done improperly. The treatment program follows a common pattern: warm-up, stretch, eccentric exercises, stretch, and ice application. Because of the difficulty (and discomfort) in applying ice in some cases, it may be omitted if desired.

Muscle tightness appears to be especially at fault in these injuries, since soccer and hockey players are, in our experience, notoriously inflexible. Hip flexors and adductors should be tested for tightness (Fig. 7.9), and special emphasis laid on flexibility exercises during treatment.

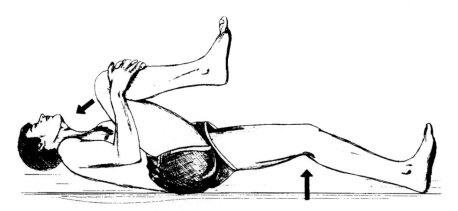

**Fig. 7.9 Testing for hip flexor tightness. Flex one knee to the chest. If the other leg lifts from the bed, the hip flexors are tight.**

Surgery should be reserved as a last resort in cases of groin injury. The two surgical approaches to chronic adductor injury are tenotomy (Martens *et al.* 1987; Akermark and Johansson 1992) and local excision of degenerative areas of tendon with side-to-side repair (Renstrom 1992; Karlsson *et al.* 1994). Good results have been reported with both types of procedures; however, the return rate to previous activity has been reported at 60–70%, which is low for an athletically active population. In addition, Akermark and Johansson (1992) have reported isokinetic adductor strength deficits post-tenotomy compared to the uninjured leg. Whether these deficits were the cause of the injury in the first place, or were as a result of tenotomy is not clear, but a strength deficit in a muscle already demonstrated to be at risk for overload injury surely cannot be a good thing. As stated previously, the post surgical rehabilitation is probably as important as the surgery, and every effort should be made to strengthen the muscle so it can withstand the demands placed upon it.

Hamstrings pull

The hamstrings, namely the biceps femoris, semi-tendinosus, and semi-membranosus (Fig. 7.10), originate on the ischial tuberosity and insert on the

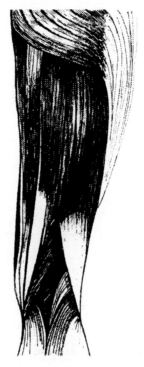

**Fig. 7.10 Hamstring muscles at the back of the thigh.**

tibia and fibula. They flex the knee, can act in hip extension, and are stretched by flexing the hip with the knee straight. During lower limb motion, the hamstrings contract eccentrically to decelerate the leg in the last part of the swing phase of gait. This activity increases as the speed of the leg increases, as in running and kicking. Indeed, it is during explosive running activities that the hamstrings are most often injured. Hurdlers would appear to be particularly vulnerable because of the extreme stretch put on the hamstrings (Fig. 7.11); however, sprinters are injured most often. There are probably two reasons for this:

(1) Higher tensions in the hamstrings during the deceleration phase of lower leg motion in the forward recovery of the swinging limb, and (2) less attention to flexibility.

The hamstrings may also be at risk because of their intrinsic properties. The high proportion of Type II fibres found in the hamstrings, as compared to the quadriceps (Garrett *et al.* 1984) may be a risk factor as well, as Type II fibres

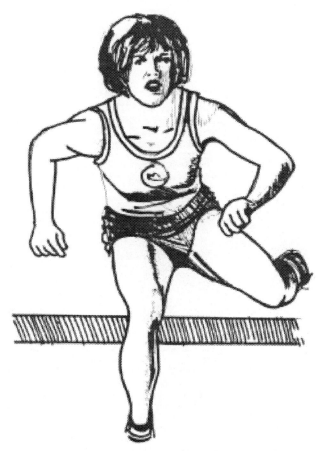

**Fig. 7.11 Hurdler showing stretch of hamstrings.**

have more intrinsic force production than Type I fibres. The high intrinsic force production, coupled with the eccentric nature of the hamstrings activation across two joints while running, appear to set the stage for high tensile strain in the muscle and tendon, and the injuries that accompany it.

Muscle imbalance has been widely accepted as a risk factor for hamstring injury. A ratio of 50–65% of hamstrings to quadriceps strength has been recommended to decrease the risk of hamstring injury (Clanton and Coupe 1998). It seems logical that the hamstrings should be of comparable strength to the antagonist muscles (quadriceps) that are eccentrically lengthening them to reduce the risk of injury. Jonhagen *et al.* (1994), found decreased eccentric hamstrings torque in injured sprinters, as compared to controls, thus underscoring the role of muscle imbalance in the pathogenesis of hamstring injury. If one accepts that hamstring injury is due to eccentric overload, and that the effects of training on muscle and tendon are specific for position, angle, velocity, and contraction type (Stafford and Grana 1984; Stanton and Purdam 1989; Friden *et al.* 1983), then it makes sense to use eccentric exercise to increase the eccentric strength of the muscle-tendon unit to decrease the risk of eccentric overload.

Treatment of hamstring injury is aimed at eccentric strengthening and stretching the muscle. The strengthening occurs as the patient lies prone and lowers a weight from knee flexion to extension, then **immediately** flexes again. This may be practised on a universal gym. Assistance may be necessary to prevent the knee from 'snapping' into extension when heavy weights are being used, or a small cushion or rolled towel may be placed beneath the ankle as it strikes the table to relieve any apprehension on the patient's part. Proprioceptive neuromuscular facilitation (PMF) techniques, combining stretching and contracting (Fig. 7.12) are particularly effective for these injuries but require a partner. As with groin injuries, special emphasis should be placed on flexibility and treatment for hamstring injuries, as decreased flexibility is associated with hamstring injury (Worrell *et al.* 1991; Jonhagen *et al.* 1994).

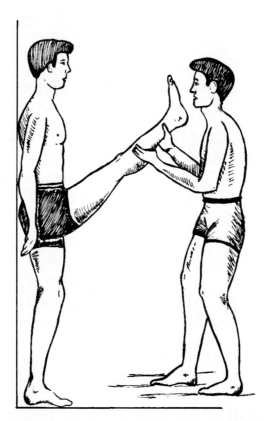

**Fig. 7.12 Stretching the hamstrings. Take leg upwards until limit is reached, then have patient try to push leg down toward bed while you resist. Then patient relaxes and you push the limb farther.**

Shin splints

**Shin splints** is a term that encompasses several different clinical entities, including posterior tibial tendinitis, anterior tibial tendinitis, anterior compartment syndrome, deep posterior compartment syndrome, and tendinitis of other deep calf muscles. The symptoms are pain in the middle one-third of the leg and tenderness along the innerosseous border of the tibia.

This injury occurs most commonly in runners who are not using properly cushioned shoes or who run on hard surfaces. It is frequently seen in tennis and basketball players also. In long distance runners, shin splints are associated with excessive forefoot pronation, that is, flat feet. This flattening of the medial longitudinal arch stretches the tibialis posterior muscle which inverts the foot and elevates the medial longitudinal arch.

Treatment for shin splints consists of reducing training mileage, anti-inflammatory drugs, local ice application, and construction of an orthotic to maintain the position of the medial longitudinal arch. Orthotics need not be complicated and may be purchased at the local drug store.

When tightness of the muscles is suspected, having the patient stand on one foot and bend at the knee, stretches the deep posterior muscles. These are the muscles that, if tight, prevent dorsi flexion of the ankle. This stretching exercise should be part of any stretching routine; it is illustrated in Fig. 4.5. The bent knee emphasizes stretching of the soleus, posterior tibial, and flexor muscles.

Tendinitis of anterior tibial muscles is commonly referred to as shin splints, but is easily differentiated because of the different location of pain. In true shin splints, pain occurs in the middle third of the leg; the pain in tendinitis of the anterior tibial muscles occurs in the upper third of the anterolateral aspect of the leg.


Compartment syndrome

The leg is divided into four compartments: the **anterior**, containing the tibialis anterior, extensor digitorum longus, and extensor hallucis longus; the **lateral**, containing the peroneus longus and peroneus brevis; the **deep posterior**, containing the flexor hallucis longus, flexor digitorum longus, and tibialis posterior muscles; and the **superficial posterior**, containing gastrocnemius and soleus muscles.

Injury to a compartment causes swelling, which can include the blood supply to the nerves and muscles contained within it. Since each compartment is bounded by a tight fascial sheath, the swelling leads to a rise in pressure within the compartment and subsequent occlusion. This is **compartment**

**syndrome**. Enlargement of the muscle without previous injury also can lead to symptoms. This usually occurs in the anterior compartment and causes impairment of function of the anterolateral muscles of the leg and of the deep peroneal nerve. The symptoms are weakness of toe extension and ankle dorsi flexion, and numbness in the cleft between the first and second toes. Compartment syndrome most often occurs in runners. It often disappears sponteneously after some time, but a favourite surgical treatment is to divide the overlying fascia (fasciotomy), thereby relieving the pressure. The results of surgery, however, are equivocle. Symptoms recur in many cases, and a loss in strength of up to 15% may occur (Garfin *et al.* 1981). Fasciotomy in cases of compartment sydrome following lower limb trauma, is considered an emergency.

## Conclusion

Therapists and physicians encounter numerous other disorders occurring in the lower limbs during sports participation that we have not discussed in other chapters of this book. In most instances, these disorders are related to trauma and so are outside the scope of this book. The cases that fall outside this classification are presented in this chapter for purposes of differential diagonsis only. Where eccentric exercise is involved, we have outlined the exercise program that should be used.

Careful history taking is important since this will tell the examiner both the injured structure and the reason for injury. Selective examination to determine the exact site of injury may be necessary and is important in isolating the muscle group at fault and exercising it correctly. In areas where several muscles perform similar functions, a non-injured muscle will perform the task, unless the injured muscle tendon unit is isolated.

Although eccentric contraction is involved in many cases of lower limb muscle injuries, particularly hamstring and groin pulls, there are equal numbers where eccentric activity is not involved. We advise you to be discriminating in applying this treatment.

# 8   Clinical results

The development of the eccentric exercise program was prompted by our disappointment with traditional treatment methods and the growing realization that we were not employing our knowledge of the behaviour of soft tissue under different physical conditions. Dr Howard Lamb, research fellow at the Nova Scotia Sport Medicine Clinic in 1978, questioned our 'standard' treatment of tendinitis, which at that time consisted of physical modalities, oral anti-inflammatories, flexibility exercises, ice application, transcutaneous neurologic stimulation (TNS), and so forth. Dr Lamb reasoned that the tensile strength of the tendon was being exceeded during activity and that this action was causing the microruptures that led to injury. Moreover, he felt that only by addressing the problem of tensile strength instability directly would it be solved. That is, the tendon must be gradually and progressively overloaded, thereby increasing its tensile strength. Immobility or disuse of the tendon (and, in fact, all soft tissues) simply weakened it. Thus we encouraged our patients to remain active, and we avoided the use of rest as a treatment modality except where absolutely necessary.

Yet we failed to take measures to strengthen the tendon. The stretching and isometric and concentric exercises that we prescribed did not produce enough tensile force on the tendon. Dr Lamb pointed this out and said we should be using eccentric loading because:

1. it simulated actual movements involved in the sport; and
2. it produced more tensile force than other forms of exercise.

Thus our eccentric exercise program was born. To examine the efficacy of the program, we surveyed 200 patients who had been treated thus. Although patients of varying types of tendinitis had been seen, we decided to review those with Achilles tendinitis, patellar tendinitis, or lateral epicondylitis because they made up the largest percentage of our patient population. The histories were documented and the diagnoses confirmed by three separate observers: the orthopedist, the research fellow, and the physiotherapist. Each patient was given specific instruction in how to perform the exercises and was checked regularly by the therapist to ensure that they were carried out correctly, and that the patient progressed appropriately.

After initial instruction, each patient was issued an instruction manual and a diary for recording daily exercise. The program was modified according to each patient's problem and the severity of symptoms at initial evaluation. We have emphasized the importance of selecting the appropriate speed of movement and amount of resistance, and this was carefully explained to each patient. Each patient's manual contained an illustrated and written description of the specific program to be carried out.

## Patient description

The group of 200 patients contained 136 men and 64 women, distributed across the three categories of injuries. Their age groups are shown in Table 8.1. The age distribution is fairly even, except for a greater number of individuals in the category of 36–40 years. This is in accordance with the higher incidence of tendinitis said to occur in the fourth decade of life. The importance of degeneration owing to aging as a likely precursor to chronic tendinitis, suggested by a number of researchers, was not apparent in our study population. The group of patients 41–50 years old had fewer, not more, individuals. Part of the reason for this may be that these individuals decrease the demand on their tendons as they scale back their activities with age.

**Table 8.1  Age distribution of tendinitis patients treated with eccentric exercise program.**

| Age group (yrs) | Number of patients |
| --- | --- |
| 10–15 | 6 |
| 16–20 | 35 |
| 21–25 | 31 |
| 26–30 | 28 |
| 31–35 | 27 |
| 36–40 | 56 |
| 41–50 | 17 |

## Symptoms

The patients were examined and diagnosed on their initial visit to the Nova Scotia Sport Medicine Clinic. At that time, a history of their current and past symptoms was obtained. The mean duration of symptoms, and secondary functional limitation, was 18 months, arranged from 6 months to 10 years. Thus, all patients clearly fell within the category defined as chronic tendinitis.

The severity of symptoms as perceived by the individual prior to the program was recorded according to this classification; mild pain with activity, not interfering with athletic performance. Moderate pain of sufficient magnitude to hinder sports activity and decrease performance. Severe pain preventing athletic performance. The number of patients in each group, both before and after treatment, is presented in Table 8.2.

**Table 8.2  Severity of symptoms in tendinitis patients before and after eccentric exercise program.**

| Level | Description | Number of patients | | Percentage of patients | |
|---|---|---|---|---|---|
| | | Before | After | Before | After |
| Mild | Pain with activity, not hampering athletic activity | 30 | 96 | 15 | 48 |
| Moderate | Pain of sufficient magnitude to hinder performance | 111 | 10 | 56 | 5 |
| Severe | Pain preventing athletic performance | 59 | 4 | 29 | 2 |
| Pain-free | | 0 | 90 | 0 | 45 |

## Sports activity

All our patients were actively involved in athletics prior to injury, except when their pain had reached a level that prevented them from participating. Even in these cases, patients were frequently involved in some activity other than that which produced their symptoms. For example, a runner with Achilles tendinitis may have switched to swimming or bicycling, or a tennis player with lateral epicondylitis may have been limited to running. We encouraged all patients to participate in sports, allowing the level of discomfort to dictate the level of this participation. Thus, the treatment program did not alter the patient's regular lifestyle. The amount of athletic activity was estimated by each patient (Table 8.3). The majority were involved quite vigorously in athletics, 80% for more than one hour daily.

**Table 8.3  Hours of athletic activity per week in tendinitis patients on eccentric exercise program.**

| Hours | Number of patients | Percentage of patients |
|---|---|---|
| <5 | 40 | 20 |
| 6–10 | 110 | 55 |
| >10 | 50 | 25 |

We examined each patient group to determine which sports were responsible for provoking symptoms. The results are presented in Table 8.4. These data support the views that Achilles tendinitis is associated with running, patellar tendinitis with jumping sports, and lateral epicondylitis with tennis. Thus, the eponyms **jumper's knee** and **tennis elbow** are, indeed, very appropriate.

**Table 8.4  Sports responsible for tendon disorder.**

Achilles tendinitis
   Running, 40%
   Jumping, 35%
   Racket sports, 20%
   Other, 5%
Patellar tendinitis
   Volleyball and basketball, 75%
   Gymnastics, 15%
   Figure skating, 5%
   Other, 5%
Tennis elbow
   Tennis, 60%
   Racketball, 20%
   Other (rare in squash), 20%

## Previous treatment

Because of the length of duration of symptoms, we expected to find that many patients had undergone previous treatment. We discovered that all patients had received some form of treatment, often more than one. On average, each patient had undergone six separate programs of treatment, with an average duration of two weeks per treatment. This confirmed the lack of success with traditional conservative treatment methods that we and others had experienced.

## Results of the program

The program sequence is as outlined in previous chapters. It is designed to be performed once daily (minimum) for six weeks. Of our patients, 20% felt that it was necessary to do the exercises twice daily.

The mean follow-up time was 16 months, so that many patients had completed the program by the time of the survey. We were able to determine the time each patient spent on the program by examining the diaries and by patient response to the survey (Table 8.5).

**Table 8.5  Time tendinitis patients spent on eccentric exercise program.**

| Time | Percentage of patients |
|---|---|
| Less than 5 weeks | 65 |
| 6–8 weeks | 30 |
| More than 8 weeks | 5 |

To determine the effectiveness of the program, we asked patients to rate their response to the program in the following way: excellent—complete relief of symptoms (44%); good—marked decrease in pain and functional disability (43.5%); poor—no change in symptoms (9.5%); very poor—symptoms made worse (2%).

Thus, nearly 90% of patients had good or excellent results, even though only 30% stayed on the program the entire six weeks. Many patients stopped the program before six weeks because their symptoms either disappeared or diminished to the point where they no longer interfered with activity. When questioned concerning their pain during sports, 45% of patients were completely normal, 48% were experiencing minimal pain without altered performance, and 7% were still hampered during athletics. The results of the program for each type of tendinitis are presented in Table 8.6.

**Table 8.6  Improvement in symptoms experienced by tendinitis patients on eccentric exercise program.**

| | Patellar tendinitis | | Achilles tendinitis | | Tennis elbow (lateral epicondylitis) | |
|---|---|---|---|---|---|---|
| | Number | Percentage | Number | Percentage | Number | Percentage |
| Complete relief | 20 | 30.3 | 31 | 54.4 | 39 | 50.6 |
| Marked decrease in symptoms | 42 | 63.6 | 26 | 45.6 | 19 | 24.7 |
| No change | 0 | 0 | 0 | 0 | 19 | 24.7 |
| Symptoms worse | 4 | 6.1 | 0 | 0 | 0 | 0 |

We can postulate that the percentage of excellent results would increase if the patients could have been prevailed upon to prolong the eccentric program for 8 or perhaps 12 weeks. This seems obvious if you make the inference that prolonging the program will strengthen the tendon even further and make it even more resistant to eccentric overload.

Those suffering from patellar tendinitis seemed to respond least well to the program; only 30% experienced complete relief of symptoms and 4% felt their symptoms were made worse. However, because of the varying lengths of follow-up, some patients were still pursuing the program and may not have reached the point where a reduction in symptoms might be expected. Since patients maintained full activity, an increase in symptoms during the first 2 to 3 weeks of the program is not unusual.

## Discussion

The results of this study are not intended to be viewed as those of a controlled clinical trial, comparing eccentric exercises with other modalities, but rather as descriptive data to assess the general efficacy of eccentric exercise plus continuing physical activity in the treatment of chronic tendinitis. Since all patients had undergone previous different forms of treatment, they would not have been suitable for a controlled trial. Our results are presented here so that the reader can see why we have been encouraged to use this program routinely in the treatment of chronic tendinitis. The advantages of the eccentric program are several. Chief among them is the fact that patients are not required to cease athletic activity during the treatment period.

   The psychological and physiologic effects of interrupting a training program are well known. For the athlete in mid-season, this interruption can be viewed as disastrous and often results in poor patient compliance. Other advantages include the following:

*Training effect*: Both muscle and tendon are increased in strength as a result of overloading.

*Flexibility*: The 'tightness' of many athletes is probably a causative factor in these, and other, injuries. The incorporation of stretching in the program promotes increased flexibility.

*Ease of performance*: The program is short and takes only about 20–30 minutes to perform. We suggest it be done at a time some hours from or (if this is not possible) prior to practice, since the discomfort from physical activity may result in the incorrect amount of resistance being applied.

*No supervision necessary*: The ability of patients to carry out the program independently saves time for both patient and therapist.

One disadvantage, in some patient's opinions, is our stipulation that ice be used after each treatment session. We feel that ice should be applied whenever possible, and if this is not readily available at the practice site, the patient should do the program at home. The major disadvantage, in our opinion, is the lack of quantification of the amount of tensile force being applied to the tendon during the variations in the exercise program. Detailed knowledge of this requires knowledge of the external forces, joint angle, muscle length, distance from line of muscle action to joint centre, speed of movement, and so on. Even when all of these forces are known, the internal state and tensile strength of the tendon will remain unknown. Until more objective information is available, we feel that using the indicator of moderate pain or discomfort at the end of 30 repetitions is a satisfactory means of ensuring that the tendon is not excessively overloaded.

As with any training program, results will not be seen immediately. This idea is readily understood by most athletes with respect to their own training programs, but may require reinforcement when applied to treatment programs. This is especially true for non athletic individuals. Ideally, the patient should be seen regularly to ensure that the program is followed correctly. Naturally, this is more important during the early stages before the patient becomes familiar with the program.

We have used eccentric exercise to great effect in the treatment of chronic tendon problems over many years. There has been little, however, in the literature regarding the use of eccentric exercise in the treatment of 'tendinitis'. The work of Alfredson et al. (1998a), discussed in Chapter 4, bears repeat mention. To our knowledge, it is the only controlled study to demonstrate the clinical benefits of eccentric exercise so clearly. The authors found that the eccentric program allowed all patients in the study group to resume full activity after 3 months, where conventional treatment failed the entire control group. Furthermore, surgery was also found to control symptoms in patients failing conventional treatment, but, most interestingly, requiring twice as long (6 months). Certainly patients will be better off if we could obtain excellent results for them in half the time and without the need for surgery.

## Conclusions

The eccentric exercise program presented in this book is one that we have used with a great deal of success in recent years. Indeed, it is our standard method of treatment in chronic tendinitis, although sometimes we incorporate other modalities as adjuncts in resistant cases. In this book, we have presented the scientific and clinical background that led to the development of the program and the results of a clinical survey that we conducted. The importance of continual progression, and careful maintenance of discomfort during exercise at a tolerable level, must be born in mind at all times. Lack of either will result, in most instances, in failure of the program.

# References
# and bibliography

## References

Akermark, C., and Johansson, C. Tenotomy of the adductor longus tendon in the treatment of chronic groin pain in athletes. *Am. J. Sports Med.*, **20**(6), 640–3, 1992.

Akeson, W., Amiel, D., and LaViolette, D. The connective-tissue response to immobility: a study of the chondroitin-4 and 6-sulfate and dermatan sulfate changes in peri-articular connective tissue of control and immobilized knees of dogs. *Clin. Orthop.*, **51**, 183–97, 1967.

Alexander, R. The mechanics of jumping by a dog (canis familiaris). *J. Zool. (Lond.)*, **173**, 549–73, 1974.

Alexander, R., and Vernon, A. The dimensions of knee and ankle muscles and the forces they exert. *J. Hum. Mvt. Stud.*, **1**, 115–23, 1975.

Alfredson, H., Pietila, T., Ohberg, L., and Lorentzon, R. Achilles tendinosis and calf muscle strength. The effect of short-term immobilization after surgical treatment. *Am. J. Sports Med.*, **26**(2), 166–71, 1998*a*.

Altchek, D. Subacromial decompression. The Toronto Shoulder Course, Toronto, Sept. 1998.

Barfred, T. Experimental rupture of the Achilles tendon: comparison of various types of experimental rupture in rats. *Acta Orthop. Scand.*, **42**(5), 528–43, 1971.

Blazina, M., Kerlan, R., Jobe, F., Carter, V., and Carlson, G. Jumper's knee. *Orthop. Clin. North Am.* **4**(3), 665–78, 1973.

Booth, F., and Gould, E. Effects of training and disuse on connective tissue. *Exerc. Sport Sci. Rev.*, **3**, 83–112, 1975.

Bosco, C., and Komi, P. Potentiation of the mechanical behavior of the human skeletal muscle through prestretching. *Acta. Physiol. Scand.*, **106**(4), 467–72, 1979.

Burton, A. Grip strength and forearm straps in tennis elbow. *Br. J. Sports Med.*, **19**(1), 37–8, 1985.

Butler, D., Grood, E., and Noyes, F. Zernicke R. Biomechanics of ligaments and tendons. *Exerc. Sport Sci. Rev.*, **6**, 125–81, 1978.

Cavagna, G., Saibene, F., and Margaria, R. Effect of negative work on the amount of positive work performed by an isolated muscle. *J. Appl. Physiol.*, **20**(1), 157–8, 1965.

Cavagna, G., Dusman, B., and Margaria, R. Positive work done by a previously stretched muscle. *J. Appl. Physiol.*, **24**, 21–32, 1968.

Clancy, W. Tendinitis and plantar fasciitis in runners. In D'Ambrosia, R., and Drez, D., Jr. (eds.), *Prevention and treatment of running injuries*. Thorofare, N.J.: Charles B. Slack, 1982, pp. 77–88.

Clanton, T., and Coupe, J. Hamstring strains in athletes: diagnosis and treatment. *J. Am. Acad. Orthop. Surg.*, **6**(4), 237–48, 1998.

Clement, D., Taunton, J., and Smart, G. Achilles tendinitis and peritendinitis: etiology and treatment. *Am. J. Sports Med.*, **12**(3), 179–84, 1984.

Coonrad, R., and Hooper, W. Tennis elbow: its course, natural history, conservative and surgical management. *J. Bone Joint Surg. (Am)*, **55**(6), 1177–82, 1973.

Cummins, E., Anson, B., Carr, B., Wright, R., and Houser, E. The structure of the calcaneal tendon (of Achilles) in relation to orthopaedic surgery. *Surg. Gynecol. Obstet.*, **83**, 107–16, 1946.

Cyriax, J. The pathology and treatment of tennis elbow. *J. Bone Joint Surg. (Br.)*, **18**, 921–40, 1936.

Daniels, L., and Worthingham, C. *Muscle testing: techniques of manual manipulation.* Philadelphia: W.B. Saunders, 1972.

Eisenberg, B., and Milton, R. Muscle-fibre termination at the tendon in the frog's sartorius. *Am. J. Anat.*, **17**, 273–84, 1984.

el-Khoury, G., Wira, L., *et al.* MR imaging of patellar tendinitis. *Radiology*, **184**(3), 849–54, 1992.

Elliott, D. Structure and function of mammalian tendon. *Biol. Rev.*, **40**, 392–421, 1965.

Enwemeka, C. Inflammation, cellularity and fibrillogenesis in regenerating tendon: implication for tendon rehabilitation. *Phys. Ther.*, **69**, 816–25, 1989*a*.

Enwemeka, C. The effect of therapeutic ultrasound on tendon healing. A biomechanical study. *Am. J. Phys. Med. Rehabil.*, **68**, 283–7, 1989*b*.

Ernst, E. Conservative therapy for tennis elbow. *Br. J. Clin. Pract.*, **46**(1), 55–7, 1992.

Fox, J., Blazina, M., and Jobe, F., Kerlan, R., Carter, V., and Shields, C. Jr. Degeneration and rupture of the Achilles tendon. *Clin. Orthop.*, **107**, 221–4, 1975.

Friden, J., Seger, J., Sjostrom, M., and Ekblom, B. Adaptive response in human skeletal muscle subjected to prolonged eccentric training. *Int. J. Sports Med.*, **4**(3), 177–83, 1983.

Fritschy, D., and deGautard, R. Jumper's knee and ultrasonography. *Am. J. Sports Med.*, **16**(6), 637–40, 1988.

Fukuda, H., Hamada, K., and Yamanaka, K. Pathology and pathogenesis of bursal-side rotator cuff tears viewed from en bloc histologic sections. *Clin. Orthop.*, (254), 75–80, 1990.

Gabel, G., and Morrey, B. Operative treatment of medial epicondylitis. Influence of concomitant ulnar neuropathy at the elbow. *J. Bone Joint Surg. (Am)*, **77**(7), 1065–9, 1995.

Galloway, M., Jikl, P., and Dayton, O. Achilles tendon overuse injuries. *Clin. Sports Med.*, **11**(4), 771–82, 1992.

Garfin, S., Tipton, C., Mubarak, S., Woo, S., Hargens, A., and Akeson, W. Role of fascia in maintenance of muscle tension and pressure. *J. Appl. Physiol.*, **51**(2), 317–20, 1981.

Garrett, W. Jr., Califf, J., and Bassett, F. 3rd. Histochemical correlates of hamstring injuries. *Am. J. Sports Med.*, **12**(2), 98–103, 1984.

Gerber, G., Gerber, G., and Altman, K. Studies on the metabolism of tissue proteins. I. Turnover of collagen labeled with proline —U- C14 in young rats. *J. Biol. Chem.*, **235**, 2653–6, 1960.

Giangarra, C., Conroy, B., *et al.* Electromyographic and cinematographic analysis of elbow function in tennis players using single- and double-handed backhand strokes. *Am. J. Sports Med.*, **21**(3), 394–9, 1993.

Gibbs, N. Common rugby league injuries. Recommendations for treatment and preventative measures. *Sports Med.*, **18**(6), 438–50, 1994.

Glazebrook, M., Curwin, S., *et al.* Medial epicondylitis. An electromyographic analysis and an investigation of intervention strategies. *Am. J. Sports Med.*, **22**(5), 674–9, 1994.

Goldberg, E., Abraham, E., Siegel, I. The surgical treatment of chronic lateral humeral epicondylitis by common extensor release. *Clin. Orthop.*, (233), 208–12, 1988.

Hutchinson, M., Laprade, R., *et al.* Injury surveillance at the USTA boys' tennis championships: A 6-year study. *Med. Sci. Sports Exerc.*, **27**(6), 826–30, 1995.

Ilfeld, F. Can stroke modification relieve tennis elbow? *Clin. Orthop.*, (276), 182–6, 1992.

Jensen, K., and Di Fabio, R. Evaluation of eccentric exercise in treatment of patellar tendinitis. *Phys. Ther.*, **69**(3), 211–16, 1989.

Jonhagen, S., Nemeth, G., and Eriksson, E. Hamstring injuries in sprinters. The role of concentric and eccentric hamstring muscle strength and flexibility. *Am. J. Sports Med.*, **22**(2), 262–6, 1994.

Jozsa, L., and Kannus, P. *Human tendons: anatomy, physiology and pathology*. Champaign, Human Kinetics, 1997.

Kalebo, P., Karlsson, J., Sward, L., and Peterson, L. Ultrasonography of chronic tendon injuries in the groin. *Am. J. Sports Med.*, **20**(6), 634–9, 1992.

Kamien, M. A rational management of tennis elbow. *Sports Med.* **9**(3), 173–91, 1990.

Kannus, P., and Jozsa, L. Histopathological changes preceding spontaneous rupture of a tendon. A controlled study of 891 patients. *J. Bone Joint Surg. (Am)*, **73**, 1507–25, 1991.

Karlsson, J., Lundin, O., Lossing, I., and Peterson, L. Partial rupture of the patellar ligament. Results after operative treatment. *Am. J. Sports Med.*, **19**(4), 403–8, 1991.

Karlsson, J., Sward, L., Kalebo, P., and Thomee, R. Chronic groin injuries in athletes. Recommendations for treatment and rehabilitation. *Sports Med.*, **17**(2), 141–8, 1994.

Kastelic, J., Galeski, A., and Baer, E. The multicomposite structure of tendon. *Connect. Tissue Res.*, **6**, 11–23, 1978.

Kear, M., and Smith, R. A method for recording tendon strain in sheep during locomotion. *Acta Orthop. Scand.*, **46**, 896–900, 1975.

Kellis, E., and Baltzopoulos, V. Isokinetic eccentric exercise. *Sports Med.*, **19**(3), 202–22, 1995.

Kennedy, J., and Baxter-Willis, R. The effects of local steroid injections on tendons: a biomechanical and microscopic correlative study. *Am. J. Sports Med.*, **4**(1), 11–21, 1976.

Khan, K., Bonar, F., *et al.* Patellar tendinosis (jumper's knee): findings at histopathological examination, US, and MR imaging. *Radiology*, **200**(3), 821–7, 1996.

Knudson, D., and Blackwell, J. Upper extremity angular kinematics of the one-handed backhand drive in tennis players with and without tennis elbow. *Int. J. Sports Med.*, **18**(2), 79–82, 1997.

Komi, P., and Cavanaugh, P. Electromechanical delay in human skeletal muscle. *Med. Sci. Sports*, **9**, 49–54, 1977.

Komi, P. Measurement of the force-velocity relationship in human muscle under concentric and eccentric contractions. *Med. Sport*, **8**, 224–9, 1973.

Komi, P., and Bosco, C. Potentiation of the mechanical behavior of the human skeletal muscle through prestretching. *Acta Physiol. Scand.*, **106**, 467–72, 1979.

Komi, P. Neuromuscular performance: factors influencing force and speed production. *Scand. J. Sports Sci.*, **1**, 2–15, 1979.

Kovalev, V. Loading—the key to jumping in volleyball. *Sov. Sports Rev.*, **16**, 99–103, 1981.

Krahl, H. Biomechanics of the human patellar tendon. In Landry, F., Orban, W. (eds.), *Sports medicine*. Florida: Symposia Specialists, Inc., 1976.

Kurvers, H., and Verhaar, J. The results of operative treatment of medial epicondylitis. *J. Bone Joint Surg. (Am)*, **77**(9), 1374–9, 1995.

Kvist, M., Jozsa, L., *et al.* Morphology and histochemistry of the myotendinous junction of the rat calf muscles. Histochemical, immuno-histochemical and electron microscopic study. *Acta Anat.*, **141**, 199–205, 1991.

Landi, A., Altman, F., Pringle, J., and Landi, A. Oxidative enzyme metabolism in rabbit intrasynovial flexor tendons. I. Changes in enzyme activities of the tenocytes with age. *J. Surg. Res.*, **29**(3), 276–80, 1980a.

Landi, A., Altman, F., Pringle, J., and Landi, A. Oxidative enzyme metabolism in rabbit intrasynovial flexor tendons. II. Studies of nutritional pathways. *J. Surg. Res.*, **29**(3), 281–6, 1980b.

Landi, A., Altman, F., Pringle, J., and Landi, A. Oxidative enzyme metabolism in rabbit intrasynovial flexor tendons. III. Changes in enzyme activity in hypovascular tendons after physical activity. *J. Surg. Res.*, **29**(3), 287–92, 1980c.

Lian, O., Engebretsen, L., Ovrebo, R., and Bahr, R. Characteristics of the leg extensors in male volleyball players with jumper's knee. *Am. J. Sports Med.*, **24**(3), 380–5, 1996.

Ljungqvist, R. Subcutaneous partial rupture of the Achilles tendon. *Acta Orthop. Scand. [Suppl.]*, **113**, 1–86, 1968.

Lochner, F., Milne, D., Mill, E., and Groom, J. In vivo and in vitro measurement of tendon strain in the horse. *Am. J. Vet. Res.*, **41**, 279–89, 1980.

Lowdon, A., Bader, D., and Mowat, A. The effect of heel pads on the treatment of Achilles tendinitis: A double blind trial. *Am. J. Sports Med.*, **12**(6), 431–5, 1984.

Lundborg, G. Experimental flexor tendon healing without adhesion formation—a new concept of tendon nutrition and intrinsic healing mechanism. *Hand*, **8**, 235–8, 1976.

MacNab, I. Rotator cuff tendinitis. *Ann. R. Coll. Surg. Engl.*, **53**, 271–87, 1973.

Martens, M., Hansen, L., and Mulier, J. Adductor tendinitis and musculus rectus abdominis tendinopathy. *Am. J. Sports Med.*, **15**(4), 353–6, 1987.

Martens, M., Wouters, P., Burssens, A., and Mulier, J. Patellar tendinitis: pathology and results of treatment. *Acta Orthop. Scand.*, **53**(3), 445–50, 1982.

Matsen, F. 3rd, Arntz, C., and Lippitt, S. Rotator cuff. In C. Rockwood and F. Matsen 3rd. (ed.): *The shoulder 2nd edn*. Philadelphia, WB Saunders, 1998.

Matthews, P. The rate of isolated segments of flexor tendons within the digital sheath. A study in synovial nutrition. *Br. J. Plast. Surg.*, **29**, 216–24, 1976.

McLoughlin, R., Raber, E., *et al.* Patellar tendinitis: MR imaging features, with suggested pathogenesis and proposed classification. *Radiology*, **197**(3), 843–8, 1995.

Medlar,R., and Lyne, E. Sinding-Larsen-Johansson disease. Its etiology and natural history. *J. Bone Joint Surg. (Am)*, **60**(8), 1113–6, 1978.

Miskew, D., Pearson, R., Pankovich, A. Mersilene strip suture in repair of disruptions of the quadriceps and patellar tendons. *J. Trauma*, **20**(10), 867–72, 1980.

Morris, M., Jobe, F., *et al.* Electromyographic analysis of elbow function in tennis players. *Am. J. Sports Med.*, **17**(2), 241–7, 1989.

Murray, M., Guten, G., Sepic, S., Gardner, G., and Baldwin, J. Function of the triceps surae during gait. Compensatory mechanisms for unilateral loss. *J. Bone Joint Surg. (Am)*, **60**, 473–6, 1978.

Nikolaou, P., MacDonald, B., and Glisson, R. Biomechanical and histological evaluation of muscle after controlled strain injury. *Am. J. Sports Med.*, **15**(1), 9–14, 1987.

Nirschl, R. The etiology and treatment of tennis elbow. *J. Sports Med.*, **2**(6), 308–23, 1974.

Nirschl, R., and Pettrone, F. Tennis elbow. The surgical treatment of lateral epicondylitis. *J. Bone Joint Surg. (Am)*, **61**(6), 832–9, 1979.

Noyes, F., Torvik, P., Hyde, W., and DeLucus, J. Biomechanics of ligament failure. II. An analysis of immobilization, exercise, and reconditioning effects in primates. *J. Bone Joint Surg. (Am)*, **56**(7), 1406–18, 1974.

Ollivierre, C., Nirschl, R., and Pettrone, F. Resection and repair for medial tennis elbow. A prospective analysis. *Am. J. Sports Med.*, **23**(2), 214–21, 1995.

Organ, S., Nirschl, R., Kraushaar, B., and Guidi, E. Salvage surgery for lateral tennis elbow. *Am. J. Sports Med.*, **25**(6), 746–50, 1997.

Ozaki, J., Fujimoto, S., *et al.* Tears of the rotator cuff of the shoulder associated with pathological changes in the acromion. *J. Bone Joint Surg. (Am)*, **70**(8), 1224–30, 1988.

Perugia, L., Ippolito, E., and Postacchini, F. A new approach to the pathology, clinical features and treatment of stress tendinopathy of the Achilles tendon. *Ital. J. Orthop. Traumatol.*, **2**, 5–21, 1976.

Plancher, K., Halbrecht, J., and Lourie, G. Medial and lateral epicondylitis in the athlete. *Clin. Sports Med.*, **15**(2), 283–305, 1996.

Popp, J., Yu, J., and Kaeding, C. Recalcitrant patellar tendinitis. Magnetic resonance imaging, histologic evaluation, and surgical treatment. *Am. J. Sports Med.*, **25**(2), 218–22, 1997.

Potter, H., and Hannafin, J., *et al.* Lateral epicondylitis: correlation of MR imaging, surgical and histopathologic findings. *Radiology*, **196**(1), 43–6, 1995.

Priest, J. Tennis elbow. The syndrome and a study of average players. *Minn. Med.*, **59**, 367–71, 1976.

Reddy, G., Gum, S., Stehno-Bittel, L., and Enwemeka, C. Biochemistry and biomechanics of healing tendon: Part II. Effects of combined laser therapy and electrical stimulation. *Med. Sci. Sports Exerc.*, **30**(6), 794–800, 1998.

Reinschmidt, C., and Nigg, B. Influence of heel height on ankle joint moments in running. *Med. Sci. Sports Exerc.*, **27**(3), 410–16, 1995.

Renstrom, P. Tendon and muscle injuries in the groin area. *Clin. Sports Med.*, **11**(4), 815–31, 1992.

Richards, D., Ajemian, S., Wiley, J., and Zernicke, R. Knee joint dynamics predict patellar tendinitis in elite volleyball players. *Am. J. Sports Med.*, **24**(5), 676–83, 1996.

Russell, A. Piroxicam 0.5% topical gel compared to placebo in the treatment of acute soft tissue injuries: A double-blind study comparing efficacy and safety. *Clin. Invest. Med.*, **14**(1), 35–43, 1991.

Safran, F., Garrett, W. Jr., *et al.* The role of warm-up in muscular injury prevention. *Am. J. Sports Med.*, **16**(2), 123–9, 1988.

Schwane, J., and Armstrong, R. Effect of training on skeletal muscle injury from downhill running rats. *J. Appl. Physiol.*, **55**(3), 969–75, 1983.

Smart, G., Taunton, J., and Clement, D. Achilles tendon disorders in runners—a review. *Med. Sci. Sports. Exerc.*, **12**(4), 231–43, 1980.

Smith, A. Estimates of muscle and joint forces at the knee and ankle during a jumping activity. *J. Hum. Mvt. Studies*, **1**, 78–86, 1975.

Snyder-Mackler, L., and Epler, M. Effect of standard and Aircast tennis elbow bands on integrated electromyography of forearm extensor musculature proximal to the bands. *Am. J. Sports Med.*, **17**(2), 278–81, 1989.

Speer, K., Lohnes, J., and Garrett, W. Jr. Radiographic imaging of muscle strain injury. *Am. J. Sports Med.*, **21**(1), 89–96, 1993.

Stafford, M., and Grana, W. Hamstrings/quadriceps ratios in college football players: A high velocity evaluation. *Am. J. Sports Med.*, **12**(3), 209–11, 1984.

Stanton, P., and Purdam, C. Hamstring injuries in sprinting: the role of eccentric exercise. *J. Orthop. Sports Phys. Ther.*, **10**(9), 343–9, 1989.

Strickler, T., Malone, T., and Garrett, W. Jr. The effects of passive warming on muscle injury. *Am. J. Sports Med.*, **18**(2), 141–5, 1990.

Suwara, R. Out of this world. *Young Athl.*, **3**, 59–61, 1979.

Taylor, D., Dalton, J., Seaber, A., and Garrett, W. Jr. Experimental muscle strain injury. Early functional and structural deficits and the increased risk of re-injury. *Am. J. Sports Med.*, **21**(2), 190–4, 1993.

Thys, H., Faraggiana, T., and Margaria, R. Utilization of muscle elasticity in exercise. *J. Appl. Physiol.*, **12**(4), 491–3, 1972.

Tidball, J. Myotendinous junction injury in relation to junction structure and molecular composition. *Exerc. Sport Sci. Ref.*, **19**, 419–45, 1991.

Tipton, C., James, S., Mergner, W., and Tcheng, T. Influence of exercise on strength of medial collateral knee ligaments of dogs. *Am. J. Physiol.*, **218**(3), 894–902, 1970.

Tipton, C., Matthes, R., Maynard. J., and Carey, R. The influence of physical activity on ligaments and tendons. *Med. Sci. Sports*, **7**(3), 165–75, 1975.

Tipton, C., Schild, R., and Tomanek, R. Influence of physical activity on the strength of knee ligaments in rats. *Am. J. Physiol.*, **212**(4), 783–7, 1967.

Vailas, A., Tipton, C., Matthes, R., and Gart, M. Physical activity and its influence on the repair process of medial collateral ligaments. *Connect. Tissue Res.*, **9**(1), 25–31, 1981.

Vailas, A., Tipton, C., Laughlin, H., Tcheng, T., and Matthew, R. Physical activity and hypophysectomy on the aerobic capacity of ligaments and tendons. *J. Appl. Physiol.*, **44**(4), 542–6, 1978.

Vangsness, C., Jr., and Jobe, F. Surgical treatment of medial epicondylitis. Results in 35 elbows. *J. Bone Joint Surg. (Br)*, **73**(3), 409–11, 1991.

Verhaar, J., Walenkamp, G., *et al.* Lateral extensor release for tennis elbow. A prospective long-term follow-up study. *J. Bone Joint Surg. (Am)*, **75**(7), 1034–43, 1993.

Viidik, A. Functional properties of collagenous tissues. *Int. Rev. Connect. Tissue Res.*, **6**, 127–215, 1973.

Wahrenberg, H., Lindbeck, L., and Ekholm, J. Knee muscular moment, tendon tension force and EMG during a vigorous movement in man. *Scand. J. Rehabil. Med.*, **10**(2), 99–106, 1978.

Walker, L., Harris, E., and Benedict, J. Stress-strain relationships in human plantaris tendon: a preliminary study. *Med. Elect. Biol. Eng.*, **2**, 31–8, 1964.

Wiemann, K., and Hahn, H. Influences of strength, stretching and circulatory exercises on flexibility parameters of the human hamstrings. *Int. J. Sports Med.*, **18**(5), 340–6, 1997.

Wilkie, D. The relation between force and velocity in human muscle. *J. Physiol. (Lond).*, **110**, 249–80, 1950.

Woo, S., Matthews, J., Akeson, W., Amiel, D., and Convery, F. Connective tissue response to immobility. Correlative study of biomechanical and biochemical measurements of normal and immobilized rabbit knees. *Arthritis Rheum.*, **18**(3), 257–64, 1975.

Wood, G. An electrophysiological model of human visual reaction time. *J. Motor Behav.*, **9**, 267–74, 1977.

Worrell, T., Perrin, D., *et al.* Comparison of isokinetic strength and flexibility measures between hamstring injured and non-injured athletes. *J. Orthop. Sports Phys. Ther.*, **13**(3), 118–25, 1991.

Wrenn, R., Goldner, J., and Markee, J. An experimental study of the effects of cortisone on the healing process and tensile strength of tendons. *J. Bone Joint Surg. (Am)*, **36**, 588–601, 1954.

Wuori, J., Overend, T., Kramer, J., and MacDermid, J. Strength and pain measures associated with lateral epicondylitis bracing. *Arch. Phys. Med. Rehabil.*, **79**(7), 832–7, 1998.

Yazici, M., Kapuz, C., and Gulman, B. Morphologic variants of cromion in neonatal cada-vers. *J. Ped. Orthop.*, **15**(5), 644–7, 1995.

Yerger, B., and Turner, T. Percutaneous extensor tenotomy for chronic tennis elbow: An office procedure. *Orthopedics*, **8**(10), 1261–3, 1985.

Zernicke, R. F., Garhammer, J., and Jobe, F. W. Human patellar-tendon rupture. *J. Bone Joint Surg. (Am)*, **59**(2), 179–83, 1977.

Zuckerman, J., and Stull, G. Ligamentous separation force in rats as influenced by training, detraining, and cage restriction. *Med. Sci. Sports*, **5**(1), 44–9, 1973.

# Bibliography

Alfredson, H., Pietila, T., and Lorentzon, R. Chronic Achilles tendinitis and calf muscle strength. *Am. J. Sports Med.*, **24**(6), 829–33, 1996.

Alfredson, H., Pietila, T., Jonsson, P., and Lorentzon, R. Heavy-load eccentric calf muscle training for the treatment of chronic Achilles tendinosis. *Am. J. Sports Med.*, **26**(3), 360–6, 1998*b*.

Almekinders, L., and Gilbert, J. Healing of experimental muscle strain and the effect of non-steroidal anti-inflammatory medication. *Am. J. Sports Med.*, **14**, 305–8, 1986.

Amadio, P. Tendon and ligament. In *Wound healing: biochemical and clinical aspects* (ed. I. Cohen, R. Diegelmann and W. Lindblad). Philadelphia, WB Saunders, 1992.

Andriacchi, T., Subiston, K., *et al.* Ligament: injury and repair. In *Injury and repair of the musculoskeletal soft tissues* (ed. S. Woo and J. Buckwalter). Park Ridge, AAOS, 1988.

Astrom, M., and Westlin, N. Blood flow in the human Achilles tendon assessed by laser doppler flowmetry. *J. Ortho. Res.*, **12**, 246–52, 1994.

Barnett, C., Davies, D., and MacConaill, M. *Synovial joints: their structure and mechanics.* London, Longmans, 1961.

Best, T., and Garrett, W. Jr. Basic science of soft tissue: muscle and tendon. In *Orthopedic sports medicine* (ed. J. DeLee and D. Drez). Philadelphia, WB Saunders, 1994.

Carr, A., and Norris, S. The blood supply of the calcaneal tendon. *J. Bone Joint Surg. (Br.),* **71**, 100–1, 1989.

Clancy, W., Jr. Tendon trauma and overuse injuries. In *Sports—induced inflammation: clinical and basic science concepts* (ed. W. Leadbetter, J. Buckwalter, and S. Gordon). Park Ridge, AAOS, 1990.

Davies, S., Baudovin, C., King, J., and Perry, J. Ultrasound, computed tomography and magnetic resonance imaging in patellar tendinitis. *Clin. Radiol.*, **43**(1), 52–6, 1991.

Enwemeka, C. Connective tissue plasticity: Ultra-structural, biomechanical and morphometric effects of physical factors on intact and regenerating tendons. *J. Orthop. Sports Phys. Ther.*, **14**, 198–212, 1991.

Enwemeka, C. Functional loading augments tensile strength and energy absorption capacity of regenerating rabbit Achilles tendons. *Am. J. Phys. Med. Rehabil.*, **71**, 31–8, 1992.

Enwemeka, C., Cohen-Kornberg, E., *et al.* Biomechanical effects of three different periods of GaAs laser photostimulation on tenotomized tendons. *Laser Ther.*, **6**, 181–8, 1994.

Ferretti, A., Papandrea, P., and Conteduca, F. Knee injuries in volleyball. *Sports Med.*, **10**(2), 132–8, 1990.

Frieder, S., Weisberg, J., Fleming, B., and Stanek, A. A pilot study: The therapeutic effect of ultrasound following partial rupture of Achilles tendons in male rats. *J. Orthop. Sports Phys. Ther.*, **10**, 39–46, 1988.

Fritz, R., and Steinbach, L. Magnetic resonance imaging of the musculoskeletal system: Part 3. The elbow. *Clin. Orthop.*, (324), 321–39, 1996.

Gabel, G., and Morrey, B. Tennis Elbow. In (ed.) W. Cannon, Jr. *Instructional course lectures Volume 47.* Park Ridge, AAOS, 1998.

Gamble, J. *The musculoskeletal system: physiological basics.* New York, Raven Press, 1988.

Gann, N. Ultrasound: current concepts. *Clin. Management.*, **11**, 64–9, 1991.

Garrett, W. Jr., and Lohnes, J. Cellular and matrix response to mechanical injury at the myotendinous junction. In *Sports-induced inflammation: clinical and basic science concepts* (ed. W. Leadbetter, J. Buckwalter, S. Gordon). Park Ridge, AAOS, 1990.

Gelberman, R., Goldberg, V., *et al.* Tendon. In *Injury and repair of the musculoskeletal soft tissues.* (ed. S. Woo, and J. Buckwalter). Park Ridge, AAOS, 1988.

Hennig, E., Rosenbaum, D., and Milani, T. Transfer of tennis racket vibrations onto the human forearm. *Med. Sci. Sports Exerc.*, **24**(10), 1134–40, 1992.

Hess, G., Capiello, W., Poole, R., and Hunter, S. Prevention and treatment of overuse tendon injuries. *Sports Med.*, **8**, 371–84, 1989.

Heyse-Moore, G. Resistant tennis elbow. *J. Hand Surg. (Br)*, **9**(1), 64–6, 1984.

Houglum, P. Soft tissue healing and its impact on rehabilitation. *J. Sports Rehab.*, **1**, 19–39, 1992.

Leach, R., Schepsis, A., and Takai, H. Long-term results of surgical management of Achilles tendinitis in runners. *Clin. Orthop.*, (282), 208–12, 1992.

Leadbetter, W. Cell-matrix response in tendon injury. *Clin. Sports Med.*, **11**(3), 533–78, 1992.

Lineger, J., and West, L. Epidemiology of soft-tissue/musculoskeletal injury among US Marine recruits undergoing basic training. *Mil. Med.*, **157**(9), 491–3, 1992.

Litsky, A., and Spector, M. Biomaterials. In *Orthopedic basic science* (ed. S. Simon). Park Ridge, AAOS, 1994.

Maffulli, N., Testa, V., *et al.* Results of percutaneous longitudinal tenotomy for Achilles tendinopathy in middle—and long-distance runners. *Am. J. Sports Med.*, **25**(6), 835–40, 1997.

Mourad, K., King, J., Guggiana, P. Computed tomography and ultrasound imaging of jumper's knee—patellar tendinitis. *Clin. Radiol.*, **39**(2), 162–5, 1988.

Nakagawa, Y., Majima, T., and Nagashima, K. Effect of aging on ultrastructure of slow and fast skeletal muscle tendon in rabbit Achilles tendons. *Acta Physiol. Scand.*, **152**, 307–13, 1994.

Nelen, G., Martens, M., and Burssens, A. Surgical treatment of chronic Achilles tendinitis. *Am J. Sports Med.*, **17**(6), 754–9, 1989.

O'Brien, M. Functional anatomy and physiology of tendons. *Clin. Sports Med.*, **11**(3), 505–20, 1992.

Orava, S., Osterback, L., Hurme, M. Surgical treatment of patellar tendon pain in athletes. *Br. J. Sports Med.*, **20**(4), 167–9, 1986.

Postacchini, F., and DeMartino, C. Regeneration of rabbit calcaneal tendon: maturation of collagen and elastic fibres following partial tenotomy. *Conn. Tiss. Res.*, **8**, 41–7, 1980.

Puddu, G., Ippolito, E., and Postacchini, F. A classification of Achilles tendon disease. *Am. J. Sports Med.*, **4**, 145–50, 1976.

Rivenburgh, D. Physical modalities in the treatment of tendon injuries. *Clin. Sports Med.*, **11**(3), 645–59, 1992.

Schenk, M., and Dalinka, M. Imaging of the elbow. An update. *Orthop. Clin. North Am.*, **28**(4), 517–35, 1997.

Schepsis, A., and Leach, R. Surgical management of Achilles tendinitis. *Am. J. Sports Med.*, **15**(4), 308–15, 1987.

Schepsis, A., Wagner, C., and Leach, R. Surgical management of Achilles tendon overuse injuries. A long-term follow-up study. *Am. J. Sports Med.*, **22**(5), 611–19, 1994.

Stehno-Bittel, L., Reddy, G., Gum, S., and Enwemeka, C. Biochemistry and biomechanics of healing tendon: Part I. Effects of rigid plaster casts and functional casts. *Med. Sci. Sports Exerc.*, **30**(6), 788–93, 1998.

Teitz, C., and Garrett, W. Jr., *et al*. Tendon problems in athletic individuals. In *Instructional course lectures Volume 46*. (ed. Springfield D.). Park Ridge, AAOS, 1997.

Verhaar, J., and Spaans, F. Radial tunnel syndrome: An investigation of compression neuropathy as a possible cause. *J. Bone Joint Surg. (Am)*, **73**(4), 539–44, 1991.

Woo, S., An, K. N., *et al*. Anatomy, biology, and biomechanics of tendon, ligament and meniscus. In S. Simon (ed): *Orthopedic basic science*. Park Ridge, AAOS, 1994.

# Index

abductor pollicis longus tendon injuries
103–5
Achilles tendinitis 8, 49–64, 105
  classification 53
  clinical results 117–23
  differential diagnosis 59
  eccentric exercise program 61–4
  etiology 21, 54–8
  examination 58–9
  sports involved 120
  surgery 60–1
  treatment 59–64
Achilles tendon
  blood supply 52–3
  bursae around 51, 52
  mechanics 54–5
  structure 49–51, 52
acromioplasty 100–1
adductor brevis muscle 106, 109
adductor longus muscle/tendon 106, 107,
  109
adductor magnus muscle 106, 109
age
  eccentric exercise program and 118
  humeral epicondylitis and 86
  patellar tendinitis and 67, 68
  tendon mechanics and 16
anabolic steroids 17
angiofibroblastic hyperplasia 24, 68, 83
ankle, sudden dorsiflexion 55–6
anterior compartment syndrome 114, 115
anterior tibial tendinitis 114
anti-inflammatory drugs 25, 27–8, 60
aspirin 27
athletic impingement 100
athletics 20–1
ATP (adenosine triphosphate) 35

backhand stroke
  in squash 87, 88
  in tennis 87, 88
badminton 87–9
basketball 43–4, 65, 114, 120
biceps femoris 111
bicipital tendinitis 101–2
bipennate muscles 4
blood supply, tendon 7–9
  along length 8
  bone-tendon junction 8
  effect of tendon injury 22–3
  internal vasculature 8–9
  musculotendinous junction 7
  zone of decreased 8

bone scans, in groin injury 108–9
bone-tendon junction 4
  blood supply 8
braces 26, 93
bursae 4
  Achilles tendon 51, 52
  knee 75, 76
bursitis
  Achilles 51, 57, 59
  knee 75

calcaneus bruises 59
calcification, dystrophic 24, 76, 90
calf muscles 49, 50
  excessive tightness 55
carbohydrate, dietary 16
cartilage metaplasia 24
cast immobilization 26, 30
  in jumper's knee 78
chronic tendon injury 1, 24
cold therapy 28
  see also ice application
collagen 4, 5–6
  healing 23–4
  metabolism 16
  synthesis 5
  tensile strength 9–11
collagen fibrils 5, 6
  breaking of cross-links 21–2
  effects of stress 21–2
  reorientation, in tendon healing 23–4, 26
  response to tensile force 11, 16, 19, 21
  wavy configuration (crimp) 6, 7
common extensor tendon 83, 84, 85
compartment syndrome 59, 114–15
compressive force 9, 10
computed tomography (CT) 77, 109
concentric contraction 34
  force–velocity relationship 36, 37
  two-component model 41, 42
connective tissue disorders 16
contractile component (CC) 41, 42
corticosteroid injections 27–8
  in Achilles tendinitis 60
  in bicipital tendinitis 102
  in humeral epicondylitis 93
  in jumper's knee 78
corticosteroids 16
creep 15
CT (computed tomography) 77, 109

deep friction massage 29
deep heat 28–9

deep infrapatellar bursa 75, 76
deep posterior compartment syndrome 114
deformation rate 14
degenerative changes 1, 22, 24
  *see also* tendinosis
depth jumping 82
De Quervain's syndrome 105
drop and stop motion 80
drug treatment 25, 27–8

eccentric contraction 34–5
  in Achilles tendinitis 55–6
  force–velocity relationship 36, 37
  in hamstrings injury 112
  in humeral epicondylitis 87
  in jumper's knee 69, 72–3, 74
  two-component model 41–2, 43
eccentric exercise program 43–7, 117
  for Achilles tendinitis 61–4
  avoidance of activity 47
  clinical evaluation 117–23
    patient description 118
    previous treatment 120
    results 120–2
    sports activity 119–20
    symptoms 118–19
  controlling inflammation 47
  for hamstrings injury 112–13
  for humeral epicondylitis 92–4, 95, 96
  for jumper's knee 79–82
  pain and 45–6
  speed of muscle contraction 44–5
  for supraspinatus tendinitis 100, 101
  tendon lengthening 44
  tendon loading 44
  for triceps tendinitis 103, 104
elastic supports 26
elastin 5
elbow
  epicondylitis 83–97
  posterolateral rotary instability 90
  valgus instability 89, 90
electrical mechanical delay (EMD) 37
electric stimulation 24, 29
electromyography (EMG) 90
endotenon 6, 8
endurance limit 2
energy 35–6
epicondylitis
  humeral (elbow) 83–97
  lateral, *see* lateral epicondylitis
  medial, *see* medial epicondylitis
epitenon 6, 8
estrogen 16
etiology of tendinitis 19–24
exercise 33–48
  collagen metabolism and 16
  in humeral epicondylitis 93–4
  as treatment modality 25, 30–1
  type 33–5

extensor aponeurosis (common extensor tendon) 83, 84, 85
extensor pollicis brevis tendon injuries 103–5
extensor pollicis longus 9, 10

fascicles 6
fasciotomy 115
fast twitch fibres 40
fatigue limit 2
fibres 6
fibrils, *see* collagen fibrils
fibrinoid degeneration 24, 68
fibroblasts 5, 6, 23
fibrocartilage 4, 8
figure skating 120
flat feet 114
flexibility training 122
  in Achilles tendinitis 61
  in hamstrings pull 113
  in jumper's knee 79
footwear
  Achilles tendinitis and 57
  flat 57
  shin splints and 114
  sole 57
force–length relationship 37–40
force–time curve 14
force–time relationship 37
force–velocity relationship 36–7
forearm brace 93
fractures, stress 59
fusiform muscles 3, 4
  tendon mechanics 19, 20

gastrocnemius muscle 49, 50, 51
Golgi tendon organs (GTO) 9, 40–1
gracilis muscle 106, 109
groin injury 105–10
  differential diagnosis 108
  imaging 108–10
  treatment 110
groin pull 107
ground substance (proteoglycan–water
    matrix) 5, 23
gymnastics 120

hamstring muscles 111
hamstrings pull 111–13
healing, tendon 22–4
  blood supply and 8
  electric stimulation and 24, 29
  inactivity and 26
heat, deep 28–9
heel
  elevation, inadequate 57
  lifts 60
hierarchical organization of tendon 6
hip flexors/adductors 105–6
  resistance testing 107, 108
  testing for tightness 110

hip joint pain 108
Hoffa's disease 75
hormones 16
humerus
    lateral epicondyle 83
    medial epicondyle 84
hurdlers 111, 112
hysteresis 14, 15

ice application 28, 45, 47, 122–3
    in bicipital tendinitis 102
    in humeral epicondylitis 93, 94, 96
ice hockey 106, 110
iliopsoas muscle 109
imaging
    in groin injury 108–10
    in humeral epicondylitis 90
    in jumper's knee 76–7
immobilization
    cast, see cast immobilization
    collagen metabolism and 16
impingement syndrome 99–101
inactivity 16, 26, 30, 47
inflammation 22–3
    control during treatment 47
    in patellar tendinitis 70
infrapatellar fat pad inflammation 75
infraspinatus tendon injuries 103
insulin 16
in vivo testing 31
isometric contraction 33, 34
    two-component model 41

joint
    moment 38–9
    torque 38–9
jumper's knee (patellar tendinitis) 65–82,
        105
    classification 71, 72
    clinical results 117–23
    conservative treatment 78, 82
    differential diagnosis 74–5
    eccentric exercise program 79–82
    etiology 20, 72–4
    imaging 76–7
    lesion characteristics 68–9
    signs and symptoms 69–71
    sites 67–8
    sports involved 120
    treatment 78–82
jumping 120
    Achilles tendon injury 56
    depth 82
    patellar tendinitis and 69, 70, 74
    tendon forces 55, 72, 73

kicking
    groin injury 106, 107
    hamstrings pull 111
    patellar tendon injury 20, 72–3

knee
    jumper's, see jumper's knee
    locking 75

laser stimulation 31
lateral compartment syndrome
        114
lateral epicondyle 83
lateral epicondylitis 83–97
    clinical results 117–23
    differential diagnosis 90–1
    etiology and mechanics 86–9
    imaging 90
    pathology 91, 92
    signs and symptoms 89
    sports involved 120
    surgery 94–7
    terminology 83
    treatment 91–7
length, tendon
    mechanical behaviour and 12, 13
    progressive increase in 44
lever arm of muscle 38
load, progressive increase in 44
load-elongation curve 11–12
lower limb tendinitides 105–15

magnetic resonance imaging (MRI)
    in groin injury 109–10
    in humeral epicondylitis 90
    in jumper's knee 77
massage 29
mechanics
    Achilles tendon 54–5
    humeral epicondylitis 86–9
    muscle contraction 35–40
    tendon 9–15
        effects of exercise 30–1
        length dependence 12, 13
        size dependence 11–12
        time dependence 14–15
    tendon healing and 24, 26
    tendon injury 19–21
mechanoreceptors 9
medial epicondyle 84
medial epicondylitis 83, 84–5
    signs and symptoms 89
    treatment 94, 96–7
meniscal tears 75
mesotenon 8
metabolic activity 15–17
microfibril 5, 6
moment
    arm of muscle 38
    joint 38–9
motor unit 40
MRI, see magnetic resonance imaging
muscle
    contraction
        speed of 44–5

static 33
types 33–5
elasticity 41–3
forces exerted on tendons 19, 20
spindles 40–1
tears 59
types 3, 4
work and energy 35–6
muscle-tendon unit 3
exercise and 33–48
mechanics 35–40
neurologic influences 40–1
two-component system 41–3
musculotendinous junction 4–5
blood supply 7

nerve supply, tendon 9
neurologic influences
collagen metabolism 16
muscle-tendon unit 40–1
non-steroidal anti-inflammatory drugs 27

orthotics 114
Osgood-Schlatter's disease 67, 71
overhead athletes 99
overuse syndrome 2
oxygen supply 22

Pacini corpuscles 9
paddling 102
pain 22, 45–6, 47
in Achilles tendinitis 58
classification systems 45, 46
in eccentric exercise program 45–6, 63–4,
123
in humeral epicondylitis 89
in patellar tendinitis 69, 72
parallel elastic component (PEC) 41, 42
paratenon 6
blood supply 8
paratenonitis, Achilles tendon 53
patellar tendinitis, see jumper's knee
patellar tendon 65–6
patello-femoral arthrosis 74–5
pathology of tendinitis 21–2
pectineus muscle 106, 109
pelvic pain 108
pennate muscles 4
tendon mechanics 19, 20
perimysium 7
peritendinitis 1
Achilles tendon 53
in humeral epicondylitis 90
peritendon, Achilles 51, 52
swelling 58
physical treatment modalities 25, 28–31
piezoelectric effect 24, 28
plantar fasciitis 59
plyometrics 82
posterior interosseous nerve syndrome 90

posterior tibial tendinitis 59, 114
pressure sensation 9
primary tendon bundles 6
proprioception 9
proprioceptive neuromuscular facilitation
(PMF) 113
protein, dietary 16
proteoglycan—water matrix 5, 23

quadriceps femoris muscle 65, 66
tightness 79
quadriceps tendinitis 67
quadriceps tendon 65–6

racketball 120
racket sports 87–9, 120
rectus femoris 65, 66, 109
relaxation 14, 15
remodelling phase 23–4
repair phase 23
repetitive loading 1–2
rest 25–6
in Achilles tendinitis 60
in humeral epicondylitis 93
limited 26
retrocalcaneal bursa 51, 52
retrocalcaneal bursitis 57, 59
rotator cuff degeneration 100, 101
Ruffini corpuscles 9
running 120
Achilles tendinitis and 49, 55
Achilles tendon forces 54–5
compartment syndrome 115
footwear 57
hamstrings pull 111
patellar tendon forces 72, 73
shin splints 114
rupture, tendon 19–20, 22
steroid injections and 27
surgical treatment 29, 79

sartorius muscle 109
scar tissue 29
semi-membranosus muscle 111
semi-tendinosus muscle 111
sensory receptors 9, 40–1
series elastic component (SEC)
41–2, 43
shear 9, 10
shin splints 59, 114
shoes, see footwear
shoulder (gridle) tendinitides 99–103
Sinding Larsen Johansson disease 67–8
slow twitch fibres 40
soccer players 72–3, 106, 107, 110
soleus muscle 49, 50, 51
sports
eccentric exercise program and 119–20
withdrawal from 26
see also individual sports

squash 87, 88, 103, 120
steroid injections, *see* corticosteroid
    injections
stiffness
    Achilles tendon 50
    knee 70
    tendon 12, 13
strain 12
    gauges, miniaturized 31
    rate 14
strap muscles 3, 4
stress 12
    fractures 59
stress-strain curve 11, 12, 13
    safe zone 19
    tendon injury and 21
stretch 11–12, 14–15, 43
stretching exercises 15, 44, 45
    in Achilles tendinitis 61
    in hamstrings injury 113
    in humeral epicondylitis 94, 95
    in shin splints 114
    in triceps tendinitis 103, 104
subacromial bursa 99
subcutaneous Achilles bursa 51, 52
subcutaneous Achilles bursitis 57, 59
subcutaneous infrapatellar bursa 75, 76
subcutaneous prepatellar bursa 75, 76
subfibrils 5
superficial posterior compartment syndrome
    114
supinator muscle 83, 84, 85
suprapatellar bursa 75, 76
supraspinatus tendinitis 8, 99–101, 102
surgery 25, 29–30, 123
    in Achilles tendinitis 60–1
    in groin injury 110
    in humeral epicondylitis 94–7
    in jumper's knee 79
swelling 22, 58
swimmer's shoulder 99, 102
synovial fluid 8
synovial sheaths 4, 8

taping 26
tenderness, in jumper's knee 69
tendinitis
    blood supply adequacy and 8
    definition 1
    etiology 19–24
    forms of treatment 24–31
tendinosis 1, 24
    Achilles tendon 53
    patellar tendon 68–9
tendon 3–17
    blood supply 7–9
    hierarchical organization 6
    innervation 9
    mechanics and function 9–15
    metabolic activity 15–17

structure 4–5
    ultrastructure 5–6
tennis elbow, *see* lateral epicondylitis
tennis players 120
    elbow problems 86–7, 88
    shin splints 114
    shoulder problems 99
tenosynovitis, Achilles 53
tenotomy, in groin injury 110
tensile force 9–11, 14–15
    tendon healing and 24, 26
    tendon injury and 19–21
tensile strength
    definition 1–2
    eccentric exercise and 117
    tendon 9–11, 19
teres major tendon injuries 103
teres minor tendon injuries 103
testosterone 16
thigh muscles 105–6
    testing 107, 108, 109
throwing athletes 102
tibial tubercle, enlarged 71
torque, joint 38–9
training, Achilles tendinitis and 57–8
transcutaneous neurologic stimulation (TNS,
    TENS) 29
treatment, forms of 24–31
triceps surae muscles 49
triceps tendinitis 102–3, 104
tropocollagen 5
type II fibres 111–12

ulnar neuritis 89, 90, 96–7
ultrasound imaging
    in groin injury 109–10
    in humeral epicondylitis 90
    in jumper's knee 77
ultrasound therapy 28
ultrastructure, tendon 5–6
upper limb tendinitides 99–105

valgus
    heel 55, 56
    instability, elbow 89, 90
vasculature, tendon, *see* blood supply, tendon
vasodilatation 22–3
vastus intermedius 65
vastus lateralis 65, 66
vastus medialis 65, 66
vastus medialis obliquus (VMO) 65
viscoelastic properties 14–15
vitamin A 16
vitamin C 16
vitamins, B complex 16
volleyball 65, 73, 74, 120

walking
    Achilles tendon forces 54, 55
    patellar tendon forces 72

warm-up exercises  44, 45
  in Achilles tendinitis  61
  in jumper's knee  79
weightlifting, patellar tendon rupture
    73
weights
  in Achilles tendinitis  63
  in hamstrings injury  113
  in humeral epicondylitis  94, 96
  in jumper's knee  82
work, mechanical  35–6

negative  35–6
positive  35–6
wrist extensors  83–4, 85
  injury at elbow  86–9
  pain on stretching  89
  stretching exercises  94, 95
  tendon injuries at wrist  103–5
wrist flexors  84, 86
  pain on stretching  89

X-rays, plain  76, 90, 109